RADIOLOGY SOURCEBOOK

A PRACTICAL GUIDE
FOR REFERENCE AND TRAINING

DOUGLAS P. BEALL, MD

Department of Radiology
Mayo Clinic, Rochester, MN

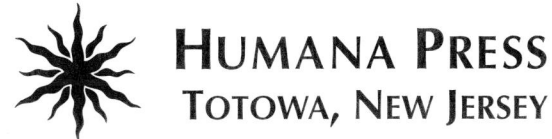

HUMANA PRESS
TOTOWA, NEW JERSEY

Disclaimer

All material published in this manual, including all clinical information, contrast formulations, sample film reporting, and technical guidelines represent the opinions of the author and do not reflect the official policy of the institution with which the author is affiliated.

Humana Press Inc.
999 Riverview Drive, Suite 208
Totowa, New Jersey 07512

www.humanapress.com

For additional copies, pricing for bulk purchases, and/or information about other Humana titles, contact Humana at the above address or at any of the following numbers: Tel.: 973-256-1699; Fax: 973-256-8341; E-mail: humana@humanapr.com, or visit our Website: http://humanapress.com

This publication is printed on acid-free paper. ∞

ANSI Z39.48-1984 (American Standards Institute) Permanence of Paper for Printed Library Materials.

Cover design by Patricia F. Cleary and Jeff Satre.

E-ISBN: 978-1-59259-287-6
Printed in the United States of America. 10 9 8 7 6 5 4 3 2

Library of Congress Cataloging-in-Publication Data

Beall, Douglas P.
    Radiology Sourcebook: a practical guide for reference and training / Douglas P. Beall.
        p. ; cm.
    Includes bibliographical references and index.
    ISBN 978-1-58829-126-4 (alk. paper)
    1. Radiography, Medical—Handbooks, manuals, etc. 2. Residents (Medicine)—Handbooks, manuals, etc. I. Title.
    [DNLM: 1. Radiography—methods. 2. Radiology. WN 200 B366r 2002]
    RC78 .B3725 2002
    616.07'572--dc21
                                                                                                2002017234

Contents

Contributors

The following have contributed to the composition and collection of information that made the publication of this manual possible:

JOHN BRIGUGLIO, MD, *Department of Radiology, of Lancaster General Hospital, Lancaster, PA*

DANIEL L. COURNEYA, MD, *University of Minnesota Medical Center, Mesabi Hibbing, MN*

BRIAN J. FORTMAN, MD, *Russell Morgan Department of Radiology and Radiological Sciences, The Johns Hopkins Hospital, Baltimore, MD*

LAWRENCE V. HOFMANN, MD, *Russell Morgan Department of Radiology and Radiological Sciences, The Johns Hopkins Hospital, Baltimore, MD*

E. PAUL LINDELL, MD, *Department of Radiology, Mayo Clinic, Rochester, MN*

THANILA A. MACEDO, MD, *Department of Radiology, Mayo Clinic, Rochester, MN*

JOHN J. SMITH, MD, JD, *Department of Radiology, Massachusetts General Hospital, Boston, MA*

PAUL S. WHEELER, MD, *Russell Morgan Department of Radiology and Radiological Sciences, The Johns Hopkins Hospital, Baltimore, MD*

ERIC E. WILLIAMSON, MD, *Department of Radiology, Mayo Clinic, Rochester, MN*

1 General Clinical Information

1 INTRODUCTION TO BASIC PROCEDURES

Early in a Diagnostic Radiology residency, many of the protocols and procedures seem foreign and can occasionally be more than a little anxiety-provoking. Despite adequate backup and supervision, all residents will inevitably have to perform a basic procedure that is not entirely within their comfort zone. The following protocols are designed to facilitate an adequate examination of the patient while giving residents a guideline to review before beginning the study. Such protocols vary from institution to institution, and they can be modified to meet the needs of the various departments using them.

Barium Esophagram/Swallowing Examination

Scout films: AP and lateral views

Upright right lateral position:

- Using video, evaluate soft palate elevation by instructing the patient to vocalize words (i.e., candy) or short phrases that cause the soft palate to move superiorly.

- Using thick barium, instruct the patient to take one swallow and visualize the oral phase of the swallowing process followed by a second swallow centering on the pharyngeal portion of swallowing.

- 2 on 1 spot film at rest.

- 2 on 1 spot film taken with the patient holding a long "e" allows the visualization of soft palate and vocal cord movement.

Upright anteroposterior view:

- Using video, instruct patient to again say a long "e". This is useful for additional evaluation of the vocal cords.

- Instruct the patient to take one swallow of thick barium and evaluate the oropharyngeal swallowing process in the AP view.

- 2 on 1 spot film at rest.

- 2 on 1 spot film after instructing patients to puff out their cheeks (i.e., like they're playing the trumpet). This provides improved visualization of the oropharynx and allows evaluation of motor abnormalities.

Upright left posterior oblique:

- Using video and thick barium, instruct the patient to swallow once. Focus on the esophagus, and follow the bolus into the stomach while evaluating the esophageal stripping waves and esophageal appearance/patency.
- Using air crystals and thick barium, take a 2 on 1 spot film of the esophagus for the evaluation of the esophageal mucosa.

Prone right anterior oblique:

- Using video and thin barium, instruct the patient to take one swallow, and follow bolus to the stomach while evaluating the esophageal stripping wave.
- Using thin barium, take a 2 on 1 spot film with the patient drinking over a bolster. This view is optimal for the demonstration of a Schatzki's ring.

Supine:

- Fluoroscopic evaluation while checking for reflux (maneuvers such as having the patient cough, Valsalva, or perform a straight leg raise are helpful).

Upright left posterior oblique:

- Take a 1 on 1 for evaluation of the stomach.

In addition to the items listed above, evaluation should include but not be limited to the:

1. Integrity of the posterior pharyngeal stripping wave.
2. Evaluation of cricopharyngeal prominence.
3. Presence of nasopharyngeal regurgitation.
4. Adequacy of laryngeal elevation.
5. Presence of adequate epiglottic tilt/cricoid motility.
6. Presence of aspiration/cough.
7. Ability of the patient to clear the aspirated material if this occurs.
8. Retention of barium in the vallecula after swallowing (pooling).
9. Adequacy of oromotor function.

Double-Contrast Upper GI

Upright left posterior oblique:

- Give gas crystals followed by a small amount of water, fluoro for position, then have the patient take 3–4 rapid swallows of thick barium while holding the barium cup in his/her left hand.
- 3 on 1 air esophagram views to include the gastroesophageal junction. Have the patient finish the reminder of the barium (if any).
- Face patient toward the table, and bring table to a horizontal position with the patient prone. Position the patient in a left lateral position and then supine.

Supine:

- 1 on 1 spot film of the stomach.

Right posterior oblique:

- 1 on 1 spot film (Schatzki view) of the gastric body and lesser curvature.

Right lateral:

- 1 on 1 spot film focusing on the anterior gastric wall, the gastroesophageal junction, and the duodenal bulb.

Left posterior oblique:

- 1 on 1 film centered on the gastric antrum.
- 2 on 1 film of the duodenal bulb (wait for air within a noncontracted bulb).

Prone:

- Place a bolster under the patient, and take 1 on 1 film of the gastric body and antrum.

Right anterior oblique:

- 2 on 1 spot film of the duodenal bulb, duodenal C-sweep, and distal gastric antrum.
- Use thin barium to obtain a 3 on 1 drinking esophagus with the bolster placed under the patient. This view should include the gastroesophageal junction.

Supine:

- Fluoroscopic evaluation checking for reflux (using cough, Valsalva, or straight leg raise techniques).

Upright left posterior oblique (LPO):

- 1 on 1 film of the gastric fundus.
- 4 on 1 spot film of the duodenal bulb and gastric antrum (with compression).

Upright anteroposterior:

- 4 on 1 film evaluation of the stomach (with compression).

Overhead Films (optional):

- AP, LPO.

NOTES

1. Glucagon (0.1 mg iv push over 30 s) can be given prior to the exam to slow gastric emptying.
2. If air-filled duodenal bulb is difficult to obtain, try turning the patient to a left anterior oblique position from the LPO position (to empty the barium from the duodenal bulb) and then back to the LPO position for the spot film.

Single-Contrast Upper GI

Prone right anterior oblique:

- 3 on 1 drinking esophagus to include the gastroesophageal junction.
- 1 on 1 spot film of the gastric body and antrum.
- 2 on 1 film of the duodenal bulb and C-sweep with compression.

Right posterior oblique:

- 1 on 1 spot film of the gastric body and lesser curve. This view should include the gastroesophageal junction.
- 4 on 1 spot film of the duodenal bulb.

Supine:

- 1 on 1 film of the stomach.
- Fluoroscopic evaluation checking for gastroesophageal reflux.

Semierect:

-4 on 1 spot film of the stomach from fundus to inferior antrum using compression.

-1 on 1 film of the gastric fundus (including the gastroesophageal junction).

Supine left posterior oblique:

-2 on 1 film of the duodenal bulb and gastric antrum. Attempt to obtain an air-filled view of the bulb if possible.

Notes

1. Glucagon (0.1 mg iv push over 30 s) can be given before the exam to slow gastric emptying.

Pediatric Upper GI

Left lateral and anteroposterior:

-2 on 1 spot film of esophagus.

-Use video fluoroscopy to examine the drinking esophagus with attention to the nasopharynx, larynx, and pharynx as well as the esophagus.

-Intermittent pausing may be necessary for the stomach to empty. A stomach distended with barium can obscure the fourth portion of the duodenum/ligament of Treitz region.

Right lateral or right anterior oblique:

-4 on 1 duodenal bulb view. Contrast should be followed from the stomach (as seen on lateral view) to the duodenal bulb and into the second portion of the duodenum.

Anteroposterior:

-1 on 1 film of the stomach, C-loop, and distal duodenum (contrast should be documented passing into the small bowel to the left of the left lumbar pedicles).

-Fill the stomach and look for gastroesophageal reflux (optimally, the child should not be crying during this part of the examination). Water siphon test should be considered if the study is primarily to exclude significant gastroesophageal reflux.

Overhead films (optional):

-One anteroposterior abdominal film to include stomach and small bowel.

Notes

1. Collimation and a conscious attempt to keep the radiation dosage to a minimum are of paramount importance in pediatric fluoroscopy.
2. The above examination should be tailored on a case by case basis to answer pertinent clinical questions.

Small Bowel Series

1. Begin with 2 cups of thin barium or dedicated "see-through" barium sulfate suspensions (or have the patient drink an additional 1 cup of barium after an upper GI series). The patient should drink the barium promptly, and a right lateral decubitus position can be used to facilitate gastric emptying if necessary. At this point a kidneys, ureter, and bladder exam (KUB)

can be taken for evaluation of the stomach and proximal-most small bowel.

2. A second KUB should be taken 20 min after the patient begins drinking.
3. Obtain follow-up films as needed. Spot film evaluation should consist of 1 on 1 films of any abnormal small bowel loops and a 2 on 1 spot film of the terminal ileum (with compression). Additionally, 1 on 1 films should be taken in all four quadrants of the abdomen. Normal transit time to the terminal ileum is between 45 and 90 min.
4. Prone angled overhead views taken with the patient over a bolster can be used to separate pelvic loops of small bowel. Another method used to separate loops of small bowel in the pelvis involves placing the patient prone and inflating the balloon under the pelvis while he or she is in Trendelenburg.

Enteroclysis

ENTEROCLYSIS TUBE PLACEMENT

1. Informed consent should be obtained and the risks/potential complications explained to the patient (risk of bowel rupture, mucosal damage, hemorrhage).
2. Test the integrity of the integrity of the tube's balloon.
3. Check the length of a stiff guidewire in relation to the length of the tube.
4. Swab the nasal passage with viscous lidocaine and have the patient sniff the gel into the nasal passage. Spray the patient's throat with lidocaine spray.
5. Warm the enteroclysis tube with warm water to soften it, and then lubricate the tube with lidocaine gel. Position the patient upright or semi-upright with the neck flexed, and advance the tube through the nose into the nasopharynx. Have the patient drink water through a straw or suck on flavored swabs to facilitate the entry of the tube into the proximal esophagus. If the patient begins coughing or gasping, withdraw the catheter into the nasopharynx and attempt to advance it under fluoroscopic guidance. This is done by turning the patient to a lateral position and directing the tube past the epiglottis while monitoring the process under fluoroscopy.
6. Position the patient semi-upright in an LPO position, and advance the catheter along the greater curvature of the stomach until the tip reaches the pylorus.
7. Insert the wire into the tube, and advance it to within 6 cm of the catheter tip. This is done to maintain the position of the catheter along the greater curvature of the stomach. Slide the tube over the wire and into the duodenum with the patient supine or in a right posterior oblique position. Keeping the wire stationary, advance the catheter tip past the ligament of Treitz.
8. Air may be injected into the stomach to define anatomy. Limit fluoroscopy time to 15 min or less if possible. In difficult cases, if the tube is left near the pylorus, it may pass into the duodenum on its own. Having the patient suck on flavored swabs can facilitate peristalsis.

ENTEROCLYSIS PROTOCOL

1. Inflate the catheter balloon with approximately 20 mL of air to prevent reflux of methylcellulose. This is an emetic and can cause vomiting if a significant amount refluxes into the stomach.

2. Inject approximately 200–250 mL of barium (see below) into the tube using 50–60-mL syringes while making sure to inject through the correct port. Visualize the lead point of the barium column, and adjust the total volume of barium injected so that the amount is enough to push the leading edge of the barium across the patient's left sacroiliac joint.
3. Inject approximately 750–1000 mL of methylcellulose at a rate of 50–100 mL/min, and take 1 on 1 spot films of distended small bowel loops.
4. Overheads: KUB and bilateral oblique films. If the patient has an ostomy, a lateral view of the ostomy should be included.

Double-Contrast Barium Enema

Left lateral:

–Do rectal exam making sure to use copious amounts of gel lubrication.

–Insert enema tube tip carefully, and inflate the balloon if no palpable abnormalities were present on the rectal exam. If rectal disease is present the tube can be secured in place with tape.

Prone:

–Introduce the barium into the colon, and run it gently to the splenic flexure. When the barium passes into the proximal-most portion of the transverse colon, clamp the enema tube and drain the excess barium (if needed).

–Pump air into the colon gently, and watch for the barium to cross the spine. At this point, check to make sure no air is leaking back into the enema bag.

Right lateral:

–Place the patient in a right lateral position while continuing to pump air into the colon as gently as possible. When the barium reaches the distalmost point of the ascending colon, turn the patient to a supine position.

Supine:

–Check to make sure the colon is adequately coated with barium.

Left posterior oblique:

–Take a 1 on 1 view of the sigmoid colon before the cecum fills with barium.

Right anterior oblique:

–Take another 1 on 1 view of the sigmoid colon or go directly to overhead views if there is substantial reflux through the ileocecal valve or if the patient is having substantial difficulty holding the barium.

Upright:

–Ensure that the barium drains into the cecum.

–1 on 1 film of the splenic flexure (right posterior oblique).

–1 on 1 film of the transverse colon (anteroposterior).

–1 on 1 film of the hepatic flexure (left posterior oblique).

Supine:

–1 on 1 view of the cecum. Attempt to fill the cecum with air by putting the patient in a right posterior oblique position and/or by placing him or her in Trendelenburg

Left lateral:

–Drain excess barium from the rectum, pump additional air back into the rectum, and obtain a 1 on 1 film of this region.

Prone:

–1 on 1 view of the rectum.

Overhead films:

–AP, bilateral obliques, bilateral decubitus views, lateral rectum (with balloon deflated using a cross-table technique), prone angled view (of the sigmoid colon), and postevacuation view.

NOTES

1. Glucagon (1.0 mg iv push over 30 s) can be given if colonic spasm is present.

Single-Contrast Barium Enema

Left lateral:

–Do rectal exam making sure to use copious amounts of gel lubrication.

–Insert enema tube tip carefully, and inflate the balloon if no palpable abnormalities were present on the rectal exam. If rectal disease is present, the tube can be secured in place with tape.

–Using thin barium, unclamp the enema tube and introduce the barium into the colon.

–1 on 1 view of the rectum.

Left posterior oblique:

–1 on 1 view of the sigmoid colon. A left lateral or a left anterior oblique position may be needed to visualize a redundant sigmoid colon optimally.

Right posterior oblique:

–1 on 1 view of the sigmoid colon.

–1 on 1 view of the splenic flexure.

Supine:

–1 on 1 view of the transverse colon.

Left posterior oblique:

–1 on 1 view of the hepatic flexure.

Supine:

–2 on 1 view of the cecum to include the terminal ileum (if reflux is present). The two views should be taken with and without compression.

–Fluoroscopically survey the colon using compression along the entire length of the colon. Spot films should be taken of any suspicious areas or any areas in question.

Overhead views:

–AP, bilateral obliques, bilateral decubitus views, lateral rectum (with balloon deflated using a cross-table technique), prone angled view (of the sigmoid colon), and post evacuation view.

NOTES

1. Clamp the enema tube before each spot film.
2. Run the barium into the colon slowly while fluoroscopically monitoring the leading edge.
3. Glucagon (1.0 mg iv push over 30 s) can be given if colonic spasm is present.

Intravenous Urogram

Scout film:

–Obtain a KUB scout film and an ipsilateral oblique if lateralizing symptoms are present.

–Take tomogram scout views of the kidneys (the depth should be appropriate to evaluate the pedicles of the L1-L2 vertebral bodies). Indications for obtaining tomograms include:

–Age > 40 years

–Hematuria (at any age)

–Evaluation of renal parenchyma

–Suspicion of renal mass.

–Tomograms can be excluded from the exam protocol if there has been a recent intravenous urography (IVU) with tomograms or if the patient has had a recent cross-sectional imaging study (i.e. CT, ultrasound [US], or MRI) demonstrating the kidneys.

–If a Foley catheter is present, clamp the catheter (exceptions to clamping the catheter include prior bladder surgery or bladder perforation).

Inject intravenous contrast:

–50 mL, single kidney.

–75 mL, medium size patient.

–100 mL, large patient.

–Leave catheter in place after contrast injection, and watch for early signs of a contrast reaction (*see* Chapter 2, Section 11).

0 Minutes:

–Tomograms.

–If tomograms are not included in the protocol, obtain a single AP view of the kidneys.

3 Minutes:

–Should be timed from the beginning of the injection.

–Obtain AP view of the kidneys.

5 Minutes:

–KUB

–Attach compression device (exceptions to compression include patients with renal colic, abdominal aortic aneurysms, ureteral obstruction, and recent surgery).

10 Minutes:

–AP view of the kidneys.

–Release compression device.

15 Minutes:

–KUB with bilateral obliques.

–The oblique films should contain the kidneys, ureters, and bladder.

Delayed films:

–Films can be taken up to 6 h after injection if there is obstruction or very poor filling of the pelvocalyceal system. Techniques to improve visualization of a distal collecting system obstruction include positioning the patient in a sitting, standing, or prone position or by raising the patient into a standing position on the fluoroscopy table while monitoring the region of interest during this maneuver.

Post void:

–KUB

NOTES

1. Common variations to the above technique include:
   a. Positioning the patient prone for improved filling of the distal collecting system.
   b. Obtaining delayed films in patients with ureteral obstruction.
2. A normal nephrogram appears 1 minute after injection and peaks 3 min after injection. Visualization of contrast within the pelvocalyceal system occurs 3 min after injection.
3. Signs of obstruction include:
   a. Normal shape of the kidney on the side of the obstruction.
   b. Homogenous but delayed nephrogram with intensification of the nephrogram over time.
   c. Columnated, contrast-filled ureter.

Voiding Cystourethrogram

Scout film:

–KUB

–Empty the bladder prior to the examination. Residual urine obtained on catheterization should be recorded.

Fill bladder with contrast via gravity drainage while watching for vesicoureteral reflux (intermittent fluoroscopic observation).

–1 on 1 anteroposterior view of the partially filled bladder.

After bladder is completely filled:

–1 on 1 AP view of the full bladder.

–1 on 1 right posterior and left posterior obliques of both lower ureters.

–1 on 1 anteroposterior views of both kidneys if reflux is present.

–1 on 1 lateral view of the bladder if the study is for a suspected fistula.

Fluoroscopically visualize the urethra:

–An oblique position should be used for males.

–Have patient void around the catheter, and remove the catheter if time allows.

–1 on 1 view of the voiding urethra. The entire urethra should be included, especially in males.

Examine the kidneys and ureters fluoroscopically, looking for reflux.

Post void:

–Obtain KUB after patient voids.

NOTES

1. Catheterization techniques:
   a. Use a stiff catheter (i.e., white Silastic or clear plastic catheter) rather than a soft rubber catheter (i.e., red rubber catheter).
   b. Use as large a catheter as can comfortably fit through the urethral meatus.
   c. If necessary, lidocaine can be used by injecting 10 mL of a 1% solution into the meatus and urethra using a syringe tip or a syringe with a large-bore iv catheter (18 g) attached. The meatus should then be held closed for 5 min.

2 CONSENT

Patients should give signed, informed consent to procedures that carry a significant risk of morbidity or mortality. Procedures that may require consent include injection of iodinated intravenous contrast (CT and intravenous pyelogram [IVP]), enteroclysis procedures, imaged guided biopsies and aspirations, and interventional procedures in the Angio/Interventional lab. The radiologist should obtain the appropriate preprinted forms and fill in the extra information specific to the situation. The risks and benefits of the procedure are explained to the patient (usually in the presence of a witness to the consent), and the patient will sign the consent form if he or she agrees to the specified procedure. **In emergency situations or when obtaining consent is not possible, implied consent, according to state and/or local laws should be documented. Patients under the age of 18 need parental or custodial consent. However, patients under the age of 18 who are themselves parents may sign their own consent. Phone consents must be in accordance with state law, and a signed note in the chart completed by the patient's referring physician may fulfill the requirement for consent in some institutions.** If a procedure is delayed, some signed consents are good for 24 hours or more as long as the procedure has not changed. Informed consent is generally not needed for injection of MR contrast and may not be needed for other forms of intravenous contrast.

3 PRE-EXAMINATION PREPARATIONS

Often, to obtain safe, high-quality radiology examinations, the patient should follow specific pre-examination instructions.

Purpose of Barium Enema, IVP, and Enteroclysis Preparation

GI

Preparation cleanses the bowel, which improves barium coating and mucosal detail and decreases the likelihood of confusing food/fecal material with a mass (barium enema and enteroclysis).

IVP

Bowel preparation increases the likelihood of diagnosing small calculi and subtle collecting system pathology.

Barium Enema and IVP Bowel Preparation

The preparation should consist of any effective combination of dietary restriction, hydration, osmotic laxatives, contact laxatives, and cleansing enemas. These preparations are given with the intent of achieving a colon that is free of fecal material (except for minor mobile debris) and excess fluid or achieving a result as close to this ideal as possible. In appropriate clinical situations, preparation may be limited or omitted.

Examples of Bowel Preparation Techniques

QUICK PREP

–1 bottle of magnesium citrate

–2 Dulcolax® tabs

–1 Dulcolax suppository

–Clear liquids for 12 hours

COMPLETE PREP

–Light lunch

–2 glasses water or juice in afternoon

–1 bottle magnesium citrate (10 oz) over ice around 2 PM

–Clear liquid dinner

–2 glasses water or juice after dinner

–2 Dulcolax tablets before bed (swallow whole)

–npo after midnight except meds

–1 glass water or juice in AM

–1 Dulcolax suppository or water enema in AM

Enteroclysis Preparation

A laxative (magnesium citrate, bisacodyl, or castor oil) may be taken during the early afternoon of the day preceding the examination. The patient should have nothing by mouth after midnight before the procedure. In certain clinical situations (intestinal obstruction), preparation is omitted. The presence of feces in the colon need not preclude a good diagnostic result for the enteroclysis.

Upper GI Preparation

–To decrease the likelihood of confusing food material for a mass and to improve barium coating.

–npo after midnight except medications.

Abdominal CT Preparation

An intraluminal gastrointestinal contrast agent should be administered to provide adequate visualization of the gastrointestinal tract unless medically contraindicated or unnecessary for the clinical indication

For many indications, the examination should be performed with intravenous contrast material, using appropriate injection techniques. Abnormal findings on a nonenhanced examination may require further evaluation with contrast enhancement.

EXAMPLES OF PREPARATION FOR ABDOMINAL CT EXAMINATIONS

Best Preparation

–npo after midnight, except medications.

–500–1000 mL of contrast the night before scanning, to fill the colon

–500–1000 mL of contrast the morning of scanning, to fill the small bowel

–250–350 mL immediately preceding scanning to fill the stomach.

Adequate, Nonemergent Preparation

–npo for 6 h except medications

–750–1000 mL of contrast 2–3 hours before scanning.

Right Upper Quadrant Ultrasound Preparation

When possible, routine gallbladder and biliary tract examinations should be done with the patient fasting for at least 8 h before to the examination for adults and older school-aged children. Infants and younger children can be satisfactorily examined after a 3-hour fast.

Pelvic Ultrasound Preparation

For transabdominal pelvic ultrasound, the patient's urinary bladder should be adequately distended. For a transvaginal ultrasound, the urinary bladder is usually empty. The vaginal transducer may be introduced by the patient, the sonographer, or the radiologist. It is recommended that a woman be present in the examining room during a transvaginal sonogram, either as an examiner or a chaperone.

Women of Child-Bearing Age

All imaging facilities should have policies and procedures aimed at reasonably attempting to identify pregnant patients before the performance of any diagnostic examination involving ionizing radiation. If the patient is known to be pregnant, the potential radiation risks to the fetus and the clinical benefits of the procedure should be considered before proceeding with the study.

4 SEDATION

Radiologists often perform long imaging studies and minimally invasive procedures on anxious patients. In some situations, the patient may benefit from a mild sedative. The supervising physician or appropriate health professional responsible for monitoring the patient must be available to the patient from completion of the procedure until the patient has adequately recovered or has been turned over to the appropriate personnel for recovery care. Examples of recommended single-dose sedating agents follow.

Examples of Single-Dose Agents

Valium®	5–10 mg po
Ativan®	1–2 mg po
Demerol®	25–100 mg im
Benadryl®	25–50 mg po
Serax®	10–20 mg po
Phenobarbital	15–60 mg po
Pentobarbital	100–200 mg po
Morphine	5–10 mg im

Use with caution in patients with chronic lung disease or elderly patients. Reverse with naloxone.

Chloral hydrate (for pediatric use only)	25–50 mg/kg up to 1000 mg po

5 OTHER MEDICATIONS

CAPTOPRIL

Use 25–50 mg po (for nuclear medicine renal artery hypertension studies). Caution in the use of angiotensin-converting enzyme (ACE) inhibitors should be exercised. The patient's blood pressure must be monitored, and an intravenous line should be kept in place to allow prompt fluid replacement if the patient becomes hypotensive following ACE inhibitor administration. If the patient is currently taking an ACE inhibitor as an antihypertensive, the daily medication should be stopped at least 24 hours (preferably 48 hours) before the examination.

FUROSEMIDE (LASIX®)

Use 0.3–0.5 mg/kg, up to 50 mg iv, for nuclear renal scan or IVP washout in adults; 1 mg/kg up to 40 mg for pediatric cases. The lasix is given as soon as good filling of the dilated pelvocalyceal system has occurred. This, followed by additional imaging, will often differentiate between an obstruction to urine drainage versus a dilated but nonobstructed collecting system. If renal function is impaired or the patient is dehydrated, the response to furosemide may be blunted.

GLUCAGON

Use 1 mg iv slowly over 30 s (optional, to relieve spasm in GI tract).

METOCLOPRAMIDE (REGLAN®)

Use 10–20 mg po, 30 min to 1 h before enteroclysis (optional, to improve motility and decrease gagging).

MORPHINE

Use 0.04 mg/kg up to 3 mg iv, for initial nonvisualization of gallbladder during a hepatobiliary scan (to contract sphincter of Oddi). The common bile duct must contain radioactive bile, and tracer activity must be present in the small bowel at the time of morphine injection. A second dosage of radiopharmaceutical may be used to accomplish this. Documented pancreatitis is a relative contraindication to the use of morphine.

SINCALIDE (CCK, KINEVAC®)

Use 0.02–0.04 µg/kg iv slow push (over 3 min), 15–30 min before the hepatobiliary agent is used, to facilitate gallbladder visualization. A gallbladder ejection fraction study may also be performed using an iv infusion of 0.01–0.04 µg/kg of sincalide. The study requires activity in the gallbladder and is usually begun 60 min after administration of the hepatobiliary agent. Numerous protocols exist, but when performing and interpreting this procedure, the interpreter should adhere to the technique and the normal values validated for a specific technique.

6 RADIATION SAFETY

Radiologists should receive radiation badges every month. These are to be worn at all times and should be returned monthly. Residents are encouraged to get into the habit of routinely reviewing their monthly film badge report. This will give individuals an estimate of their degree of radiation exposure.

2   Contrast

The use of contrast material is vital to the practice of radiology. A radiologist is expected to learn to use contrast material in a safe and effective manner. Contrast material is used to enhance the conspicuity of lesions various organs, tissues, and potential spaces. Special formulations and volumes of contrast are administered in various ways, depending on the clinical situations, as is outlined below. The radiologist must select the appropriate type, concentration, volume, and mode of delivery of contrast for each clinical setting. Certain types of contrast carry increased risk for patients, in certain clinical settings. The radiologist must weigh the risks and benefits of contrast administration and choose appropriately. Guidelines for various situations are outlined in the following sections.

1 GI FLUOROSCOPIC CONTRAST

There are two major techniques of fluoroscopic bowel opacification: single-contrast and double-contrast. In single-contrast studies, dilute contrast is used to distend the lumen. Lesions are then seen as profile abnormalities, or as filling defects with compression. The fluoroscope is set to a higher kilovoltage (110–120 kVp) than is used in double-contrast studies. In the latter, the mucosa is coated with thick barium contrast, and the lumen is distended with air. Lesions are coated, and good distention is vital. The fluoroscope is set to a relatively lower kilovoltage (90–100 kVp).

There are two major types of fluoroscopic bowel contrast: *barium suspensions* and water-soluble, iodine-containing *contrast preparations*. Barium preparations can be used with both single- and double-contrast techniques. Water-soluble contrast is used only with the single-contrast technique. If there is a risk of aspiration, barium is preferred, as water-soluble contrast is hyperosmolar and may cause alveolar edema. Alternatively, a low-osmolar nonionic water-soluble agent (such as Optiray 160® or Omnipaque 180®) could be considered if a risk of aspiration exists. If there is a risk of bowel perforation, water-soluble contrast is preferred, as barium extravasation is irritating and produces foreign body granulomata and subsequent adhesions.

Adult Esophagram/Upper GI

Thick Barium (i.e., EZ Barium)

The patient can only drink thick barium by cup, not through a straw. Thick barium is good for upright, double-contrast esophagus, stomach, and duodenal views.

Thin Barium (i.e., Barosperse Barium)

The patient can drink through a straw. It is good for prone right anterior oblique drinking esophagus images. It does not coat the esophagus as well as thick barium but has a faster small bowel transit time. Thin barium is useful for evaluation of the small bowel. For evaluation of the small bowel only, the radiologist may skip thick barium and go straight to thin to speed the transit of contrast through the small bowel. Owing to suboptimal coating with the thin barium, the stomach is less well assessed.

Nonsterile Hypaque Iodinated Contrast

A water-soluble contrast material that comes in a *nonsterile* powdered formulation. It is usually mixed with tap water at 20% for fluoroscopy, or 2% for CT and is adequate for single-contrast evaluation of the stomach, duodenum, or colon. This contrast is suboptimal for examination of the small bowel because the contrast is hyperosmolar, draws fluid into the bowel, and dilutes the column of contrast, making it difficult to see. It is often requested by surgeons to evaluate possible small bowel obstruction, as barium may get impacted and desiccated proximal to an obstruction and may spill into the peritoneum if surgery is necessary. As the contrast passes through the small bowel, however, the hyperosmolarity draws fluid into the bowel lumen, diluting the contrast material. This can make evaluation of distal small bowel obstructions extremely difficult, if not impossible.

GastroView Iodinated Contrast

A water-soluble contrast material that comes in comes in *sterile*, premixed bottles and is similar to 20% Hypaque.

Esophotrast Barium or EZ Paste Barium

Thick barium paste is used to evaluate the esophagus. Similar products are available from different manufacturers. One can mix this with applesauce or put it on graham crackers.

Nonionic Iodinated Contrast (i.e., Omnipaque)

This is a sterile, nonionic iodinated contrast. It is useful for initial swallows in a patients with a high likelihood of aspiration. If aspirated, it is slightly less damaging to lung tissue. A significant disadvantage is that it has a very bitter taste, and it may be necessary to instill this contrast through a tube placed in the esophagus.

Pediatric Upper GI

EZ Paque Barium or Nonsterile Nonionic Iodinated Contrast (25–30%) if barium is contraindicated.

Be careful with Gastroview in children. It is hyperosmolar and may lower intravascular volume by drawing fluid into bowel.

Enteroclysis

I.e., Entero H Barium

Micropulverized barium preparation, which coats well. It is washed through the small bowel with large volumes of methylcellulose or water.

Double-Contrast Barium Enema

Polybar Barium

Very thick barium preparation with good coating. However, slower moving column of contrast.

AC® Barium

Thinner barium preparation with poorer coating, but faster moving column.

Example

An example of a recipe for double-contrast barium enema is 50:50 Polybar/AC. If the patient is less mobile, the radiologist may want to go to 100% AC, to improve the barium flow.

Single-Contrast Barium Enema

Examples of recipes:

1 large can Hypaque®, mixed to 1200 mL, with water, *or*
4 bottles GastroView, mixed to 1200 mL with water.

Start with 1200 mL and make more if needed, for large-volume colons.

Rectum and Pelvic Floor Examination

EZ Paste Barium

Colostomy Study

100% AC Barium; give glucagon if appropriate.

2 BILIARY CONTRAST

I.e., Sterile Hypaque Iodine (Ionic) Contrast

This comes in *sterile*, premixed bottles at 60% and is useful for opacification of the biliary tree, sinus tracts, and gastros-

tomy tubes, during fluoroscopy. This contrast will be rapidly absorbed from most tissues, including the peritoneum and connective tissues, should it end up there.

3 BLADDER CONTRAST

I.e., Cysto-Conray®

This comes in sterile, 500-mL (adult) and 250-mL (pediatric) single-use bottles and is useful for cystograms and vesicoureterograms (VCUGs).

4 INTRAVENOUS CONTRAST

Similar intravascular contrast agents are used for angiography, CT, and intravenous pyelography (IVP). All contain iodine, as the primary element for attenuating the x-ray beam. The older, less expensive contrast agents have iodine-containing molecules that are ionic. Most newer agents are nonionic. Use of nonionic agents is associated with fewer serious contrast reactions and fewer subjective complaints from patients about the injection. The newest agents, in addition to being nonionic, are also iso-osmolar to plasma. These seem to be the safest, best tolerated agents. Various formulations contain different concentrations of iodine. The radiologist can calculate the iodine content of different volumes of various agents. The radiologist should obtain consent from all patients before administration of contrast. When getting consent, one approach is to communicate to patients that "the administration of contrast is a safe and routine procedure. The benefits of using contrast, in general, clearly outweigh the risk. However, there is a small risk (1 in 50,000–100,000) of a life-threatening reaction.

A second important decision to consider is the volume of contrast to use. For older patients, smaller patients, and patients with renal disease, less contrast should be used. Under most nonemergent situations, there is a limit to the amount of contrast used. For CT and IVP, this is generally a single dose per day. For angiography, administration of more contrast is acceptable.

A third important decision to make is the contrast flow rate. This may depend on the size of the needle, the size and strength of the vein that has been accessed, and the desired bolus rate. Higher flow rates are generally better, especially for CT, but be careful not to rupture veins and extravasate contrast. Angiographers must select volumes and flow rates to opacify fully the vessels that have been accessed.

Finally, there are several others factors to consider when administering contrast. One of the most significant complications of intravenous contrast administration is the subsequent development of contrast-induced nephropathy. Intravenous contrast should only be given within the set guidelines of the department. Examples of these of guidelines are described.

Examples of General Guidelines for Patients with Normal Renal Function

If recent creatinine is less than 1.5 mg/dL, then OK to give iv contrast.

If recent creatinine is between 1.5 and 2.0 mg/dL, then give iv contrast if it is necessary to answer the clinical question. You may decrease the volume of contrast administered, as well, from 100 to 75 or even 50 mL. Also, this type of patient may benefit from hydration before contrast infusion.

If recent creatinine is 2.0–3.0 mg/dL, then get referring doctor involved in decision since the patient may get acute, irreversible renal failure and will need follow-up to assess renal function.

If recent creatinine is greater than 3.0 mg/dL, then don't give iv contrast unless referring doctor insists (and preferably provides written documentation to that effect) This patient may need dialysis after contrast infusion.

Do not administer iv contrast with a concurrent chemotherapy or blood infusion, because is there is a reaction, there may be confusion as to whether the reaction was to the contrast, or the blood, or the chemotherapy agent.

General Rules for Patients with Decreased Renal Function

If recent creatinine is less than 1.7 mg/dL, then OK to give iv contrast.

If recent creatinine is between 1.7 and 2.0 mg/dL, then give iv contrast only if necessary to answer the clinical question.

If recent creatinine is greater than 2.0 mg/dL, then get referring doctor involved in decision and don't give iv contrast unless referring doctor insists.

For a creatinine value to be relevant, it should be less than 2 months old.

Pay special attention to diabetics and other patients with medical renal disease, as well as older men with prostate problems.

If creatinine doubles over a month, renal function has decreased 50%.

If creatinine doubles over 24 h, renal function is essentially zero.

Don't forget that thinner, older patients with poor muscle mass may have a relatively low baseline creatinine. For example, a rise in creatinine from 0.4 to 0.8 mg/dL in these patients may represent a 50% loss of function. A rise from 0.4 to 1.2 mg/dL may represent a 75% loss of function. Keep in mind that the creatinine level is an indirect indicator (albeit the most clinically relevant) of renal function.

If the patient has end-stage renal failure necessitating routine hemodialysis, contrast material does not usually cause difficulties as long as the patient undergoes dialysis promptly after the exam.

Glucophage®

There is no interaction between Glucophage and iv contrast. The problem is that if the patient develops renal failure acutely because of the contrast, toxic levels of Glucophage can quickly accumulate and result in a lethal lactic acidosis.

Have patient stop Glucophage for 48 h after iv contrast injection. If the patient is at high clinical risk for renal failure, he or she should have renal function checked prior to reinitiating the medication 48 h after the examination. If the patient notices no difference in the pattern of urine production and if the referring clinician agrees that no surveillance is necessary, the patient can subsequently resume oral hypoglycemics after 2 days.

Patients with a History of Contrast Reaction

Find out what type of reaction the patient experienced. Sometimes the patients confuse the feeling of warmth associated with an injection of contrast with a reaction.

For a history of serious iv contrast reaction such as bronchospasm and hypotension, and including hives, one must premedicate the patient with glucocorticoids prior to giving contrast.

Make sure the patient was premedicated appropriately.

Always administer nonionic iv contrast.

EXAMPLE OF PREMEDICATION FOR PRIOR CONTRAST REACTION

Prednisone 40 mg po
  –Two doses: 12–18 h and 2 h before exam, *or*
  –Three doses: 24, 12, and 2 h before exam.

PATIENTS WITH

Allergy

In patients with a history of asthma or chronic hives, consider using nonionic iv contrast.

Very Poor Cardiopulmonary Function

Such patients should get nonionic iv contrast. They are at increased risk of mortality, should the contrast trigger pulmonary edema.

A Breast Feeding Baby

Previously an absolute contraindication for iv contrast; now considered safe for mothers with breast feeding infants.

Sickle Cell Disease

If the patient is in acute crisis, don't give iv contrast unless referring doctor insists, because of an increased risk of RBC sickling.

Patients not currently in crisis can receive iv contrast, at the discretion of the radiologist.

Multiple Myeloma

Absolute contraindication for iv contrast.

Possible Pheochromocytoma

Need α-blockers accessible prior to the administration of iv contrast.

The administration of contrast to these patients could potentially trigger a hypertensive crisis.

Summary of Contraindications for Contrast

Previous significant contrast reaction

History of anaphylaxis or nontrivial allergy to anything

Chronic urticaria or angioedema

Sickle cell anemia, multiple myeloma, asthma, or significant renal disease

Severe cardiac dysfunction or general debilitation.

Technique for Injection of Contrast

Check the creatinine. Obtain written, informed consent. Apply a tourniquet and gravity to distend veins. Select a contrast agent and draw up the desired volume. Select a type of needle (butterfly or angiocath) and a size (18–23 g). Connect the syringe to the needle, and expel all air from the system. Select a vein, and prep the overlying skin with an alcohol pad. Insert the needle into the vein, and tape down. For most injections done by hand, deliver the contrast as fast as you can push it through the needle while watching the vein for signs of extravasation. Palpate around the vein occasionally. A test injection with 10 mL of normal saline may be done before the injection of contrast material. Test injections are used in some institutions and may possibly reduce the incidence of contrast extravasation.

For power injection, set the flow rate (dependent on needle size)

Needle	Injection rate (mL/s)
23-g butterfly	Up to 1.5
21-g butterfly	Up to 3.0
20-g angiocath	Up to 3.5
18-g angiocath	Up to 5.0

Do a quick test injection. Deliver the contrast, and palpate the area around the access during injection. An extravasation will not always appear as an enlarging mass; sometimes it may just be a firming of the surrounding tissues. If an extravasation is detected, turn the injector off and then remove needle. Stay nearby for a reasonable amount of time to confirm that no contrast reaction has occurred.

Examples of IV Contrast Agents for CT

Omnipaque 350: 150, 125, 100, or 75 mL

Nonionic. Low incidence of contrast reaction, causes less tissue damage with extravasation. Higher cost.

Ultravist 300®: 150, 125, 100, or 75 mL

Similar to Omnipaque 350.

Examples of IV Contrast Agents for IVP

Ultravist 300/Omnipaque 350: 150, 100, or 75 cc

Nonionic. Lower incidence of contrast reaction. Causes less tissue damage with extravasation. Higher cost. Image quality slightly inferior to Conray 400®, with IVP.

Sterile 60 % Hypaque

Ionic. Slightly lower iodine concentration than Conray 400.

Conray 400

Ionic. Highest iodine concentration. Good image quality. Less expensive. Higher incidence of contrast reaction than nonionics. Causes more tissue damage with extravasation.

Reno-M-60®

Ionic. Similar to Conray.

5 ORAL CONTRAST FOR CT

Dilute barium, or water-soluble iodinated contrast, is given by mouth to opacify the bowel before CT scanning. This contrast can be made in several ways. One of the most common formulations is 3% Hypaque in water, or clear juice. This can be made by mixing:

- −3 scoops (10 g/scoop) of Hypaque sodium powder in 1.5 L of water or juice
- −2 vials (10 g/vial) Hypaque sodium powder in 1.5 L of water
- −Oral contrast material can also be purchased as a ready-to-use barium sulfate suspension (i.e., Prepcat®). These formulations commonly contain 1.5% barium sulfate along with flavoring agents such as sorbitol and citric acid simethicone.

The type of contrast, the volume, and the amount of time needed before scanning varies. For routine body CT scanning, an example of an oral contrast protocol is:

- −npo after dinner
- −750 mL of contrast before bed to fill the colon
- −750 mL of contrast 60–90 min before scanning.

The ideal is rarely the reality. In most situations, the patient is given 1.5 L of contrast, over 15–30 minutes, and then scanned 1–3 hours later. For emergent studies, use oral contrast only when indicated and wait as long as is necessary. In cases of trauma, you probably just need to get the study done as quickly as possible. Other special situations are included in *Table 1*.

Table 1
Examples of Oral Contrast Protocols

Area of interest	Contrast type/amount	Waiting time
Entire bowel	1 large cup (1000 mL) of oral contrast	2–3 h
Esophagus	2 teaspoons of esophageal paste contrast	Immediately
Pancreas	2 large cups of water	Immediately
Biliary system	2 large cups of water	Immediately
CT angiography	2 large cups of water	Immediately
Small bowel	1 cup (750 mL) of oral contrast	45–60 min
Terminal ileum	1 cup (750 mL) of oral contrast	90 min
Sigmoid colon	1 large cup (1000 mL) of iodinated oral contrast	2–3 h
Rectum	200–300 mL of contrast via rectal tube	Immediately

6 BLADDER CONTRAST FOR CT

Use diluted bladder contrast (i.e., Cysto-Conray) decreased in concentration to a 3% solution. Instill via Foley catheter via gravity. Can also use Hypaque-60 or Reno-M-60 diluted 1:10 with saline.

7 INTRATHECAL CONTRAST FOR CT

Nonionic, iodinated contrast is instilled intrathecally through a spinal needle prior to CT myelography. Examples of myelography preparations and volumes are as follows:

15 mL of Omnipaque 180

12 mL of Omnipaque 240

10 mL of Omnipaque 300

Ionic contrast is *absolutely contraindicated,* **owing to the risk of seizures and other serious complications. Always double check the contrast administered intrathecally to make sure it is** *nonionic.*

8 MR CONTRAST

Contrast material is also given for MR examinations. The vast majority of these agents contain gadolinium. The two major categories of MR contrast are the general purpose agents and the organ- or tissue-specific agents. The other categories, including oral MR contrast and the non-[^{1}H] contrast agents, will not be addressed in this section.

General Purpose Agents

Gadopentetate (Gd-DTPA), *Magnevist*® (469 mg/mL)
– Standard dose: 0.1 mmol/kg or 0.2 mL/kg
– Dose range: 0.05–0.3 mmol/kg

Gadoteridol (Gd-HP-DO3A), *ProHance*® (279.3 mg/mL)
– Standard dose: 0.1 mmol/kg or 0.2mL/kg
– Dose range: 0.05–0.3 mmol/kg

Gadodiamide (Gd-DTPA-BMA), *Omniscan* (287 mg/mL)
– Standard dose: 0.1 mmol/kg or 0.2 mL/kg
– Dose range: 0.05–0.3 mmol/kg

Gadodiamide (Gd-DTPA-BMA), *Dotarem*® (279.3 mg/mL)
– Standard dose: 0.1 mmol/kg or 0.2 mL/kg
– Dose range: 0.1–0.3 mmol/kg

Gadobenate Dimeglumine (Gd-BOPTA), Multihance®
(334 mg/mL)
– Standard dose: 0.05–0.1 mmol/kg or 0.1–0.2 mL/kg
– Dose range: 0.05–0.2 mmol/kg

Note: The hepatic uptake of Gd-BOPTA is 3–5%, and liver enhancement is noted up to 2 hours post injection. This gadolinium-based contrast is therefore useful as an extracellular agent in the first few minutes after injection as well as a hepatic agent when acquiring delayed images.

Organ/Tissue-Specific Agents

T1 AGENTS

Gadobenate dimeglumine (Gd-BOPTA), *Multihance*
(334 mg/mL)
– Standard dose: 0.05–0.1 mmol/kg or 0.1–0.2 mL/kg

– Dose range: 0.05–0.2 mmol/kg
– This agent initially distributes in the extracellular fluid and behaves like Gd-DTPA. The hepatic uptake produces sustained T1 enhancement and allows delayed images of the liver to be obtained 1–2 hours later

Gadoxetic acid disodium (Gd-EOB-DTPA), *Eovist**
(181 mg/mL)
– Standard dose: 0.025 mmol/kg or 0.1 mL/kg
– Dose range: 0.025 mmol/kg or 0.1 mL/kg (only approved dose)
– Eovist also shows immediate extracellular fluid distribution, but approximately 50% of this agent is extracted by hepatocytes. Maximum contrast between normal and abnormal hepatic tissue occurs 20–45 min after injection (imaging time range is about 2 h). A substantial portion of this contrast is also excreted in the bile and can be seen as positive contrast enhancement on the postinjection images.

*At the time of publication, Eovist was not yet FDA-approved.

Mangafodipir trisodium (Mn-DPDP), *Teslascan*®
(37.9 mg/mL)
– Standard dose: 0.1 mL/kg (5 µmol/kg) infused at 2–3mL/min up to a total volume of 15 mL
– Teslascan is not a liver-specific agent but is manganese-based and is taken up by tissues that are rich in mitochondria. This agent is taken up in the liver, kidneys, adrenals, pancreas, myocardium, and gastrointestinal mucosa. The manganese produces T1 enhancement in the liver for several hours after the injection, with an optimal imaging window of 20 min to 4 h (abnormal retention of contrast may be further emphasized on 24-h delayed images).

T2 AGENTS

Ferumoxides: AMI-25®*, Feridex*®*, Endorem*® (mean particle size 150 nm)
– Standard dose: 10 mmol/kg or 11.2 mg of Fe/mL (and 61.3 mg of mannitol)

–Dose range: 7.5–15 mmol/kg

–The ferumoxides are administered as a dilute infusion (i.e., with 100 mL D5W) over 30 min to minimize adverse reactions, especially back pain.

–Particles are taken up by the reticuloendothelial cells of the liver, spleen, and bone marrow, with about 80% of the dose reaching the liver in normal patients. Because of the magnetic field inhomogeneity induced by these agents, the liver appears dark on both T1- and T2-weighted images. Optimal images are obtained 30–120 min after injection.

–These agents are contraindicated in patients with hemochromatosis or a hypersensitivity to iron.

Ferucarbotran (SHU555A), Resovist® (mean particle size 60 nm)

–Standard dose: 8 mmol/kg

–Dose range: 8–10 mmol/kg

–Resovist may be given by a rapid bolus injection. A T1 enhancement is observed for the first few minutes after injection, but the agent is then taken up by the reticuloendothelial cells, causing significant T2 shortening (similar to the ferumoxides). Because of the T1 enhancement, Resovist produces dynamically enhanced images that are analogous to gadopentate.

–The T2 agents listed above are effective at all magnetic field strengths but produce the greatest effect with stronger magnetic fields.

9 IODINATED CONTRAST FORMULATIONS

Trade name	Iodine content (mg/mL)	Trade name	Iodine content (mg/mL)
Angiovist 282, 292, 370®	282, 292, 370	**Optiray**® * 160, 240, 320	160, 240, 320
Conray 30, 43, 325, 400®	141, 202, 325, 400	Renografin 60, 76®	292, 370
Conray® (plain), Cysto-, Angio-	282, 81, 480	Reno-M DIP, 60®	141, 282
Diatrizoate meglumine 76%	358	Reno-M-60®	282
GastroView®	367	Renovue DIP, 65®	111, 300
Hexabrix® **	320	Renovist II®	309
Hypaque Meglumine® 30%, 60%	141, 282	Renovist®	370
Hypaque Sodium® 25%, 50%	150, 300	**Ultravist 300**®*	150, 240, 300, 370
Hypaque-76®	370	Urovist Meglumine® (Cysto-141)	141
Hypaque-M® 75%, 90%	385, 462	Urovist Sodium 300®	300
Isovue® * 128, 200, 300, 370	128, 200, 300, 370	Vascoray®	400
MD 60, 76®	292, 370	*Nonionic.	
Omnipaque® * 180, 240, 300, 350	180, 240, 300, 350	**Low osmolality, but ionic.	

10 CONTRAST EXTRAVASATION AND TREATMENT

Contrast extravasation into the soft tissue surrounding the injection site is a relatively common complication of examinations involving iv contrast injection. The severity of this complication can range from trivial to limb-threatening. Examples of treatment for this untoward event are described.

Minimal Extravasation

> 5 mL

No treatment or follow-up needed.

Moderate Extravasation

< 30 mL ionic or < 100 mL nonionic

Elevation of arm above heart

Watch patient for 2–4 h

Call referring physician

Ice packs three times per day for 1–3 days

Document extravasation

Have patient call referring physician if problem arises.

Marked Extravasation

> 30 mL ionic or > 100 mL nonionic

Immediate surgical (i.e., plastic surgery) consultation

Assess for:

–Skin blistering

–Altered tissue perfusion distal to site of extravasation

–Change in sensation distal to site of extravasation

–Increasing pain after 2–4 h.

Document extravasation and notify risk management

Daily phone calls by nurse or radiologist until problems resolve.

11 CONTRAST REACTIONS AND TREATMENT

Check ABCs and vital signs.

Urticaria, Pruritis, or Erythema

Mild to moderate

No therapy needed in most cases.

Benadryl 50 mg or 1 mg/kg po/im/iv

Watch for 30 min

Have someone drive the patient home.

Severe

Epinephrine 1:1000, 0.3 mL sq, or 0.01 mL/kg, if no cardiac contraindication.

Facial or Laryngeal Edema, or Stridor

Oxygen

Epinephrine 1:1,000, 0.3 mL sq (0.01 mL/kg)

  –If sq epinephrine fails or if patient experiences vascular collapse, then give *epinephrine* 1:10,000 3 mL iv slow push.

Bronchospasm or Wheezing

Oxygen, pulse oximeter (severe, < 88%)

Bronchodilator nebulized in NS 2.5 mL, such as:
  –Isoetharine 1% [Bronkosol®] 0.25–0.5 mL
  –Albuterol 0.5% [Ventolin®, Proventil®] 0.5 mL
  –Metaproterenol 5% [Alupent®, Metaprel®] 0.3 mL

If no improvement: *epinephrine* 1:1000, 0.3 mL sq (0.01 mL/kg)

If sq fails or if patient experiences vascular collapse then give: *epinephrine* 1:10,000, 3 mL iv slow push.

Hypotension

With Tachycardia, or Shock

Oxygen, Trendelenberg

Lactated Ringer's Solution, iv wide open

If no improvement: *epinephrine* 1:1000, 0.3 mL sq (0.01 mL/kg)

If sq fails or vascular collapse: *epinephrine* 1:10,000, 3 mL iv slow push.

With Bradycardia (Vagal Reaction): no β-Blocker

Oxygen, Trendelenberg

Lactated Ringer's Solution, iv wide open

If no improvement: *atropine* 0.5–1.0 mg iv slow push, repeat up to 2.0 mg total.

3 Common Procedures

1 BASIC ABDOMINAL IMAGE-GUIDED INTERVENTION

The advent of CT and ultrasound (US) has provided dramatically improved diagnostic accuracy as well as expanded capabilities for image-guided therapy. Image-guided interventions within the abdomen and retroperitoneum are numerous and include abscess drainage, tumor biopsy, biliary intervention, and percutaneous nephrostomy tube placement.

The mortality associated with an undrained abscess is significant, and some authors have reported rates approaching 100%. Historically, surgical abscess drainage has been the mainstay of intraabdominal abscess treatment, but more recently image-guided abscess drainage techniques have offered comparable successrates, and lower morbidity/mortality rates.

Both CT and US are highly effective at detecting intraabdominal malignancies and can be used for percutaneous image-

guided tissue sampling of these masses. Traditionally, only US has provided real-time intervention guidance, but, with the development of fluoroscopy capability, CT can now do the same thing. Real-time guidance has the potential to reduce procedure time, to facilitate placement of the needle or catheter into the appropriate position, and to improve procedural efficacy.

Needles, Catheters, Drains, and Miscellaneous Equipment

The equipment set used for various interventional procedures within the abdomen and retroperitoneum will vary widely according to the specific procedure. Various types of equipment used in such interventions are listed below. This is neither an

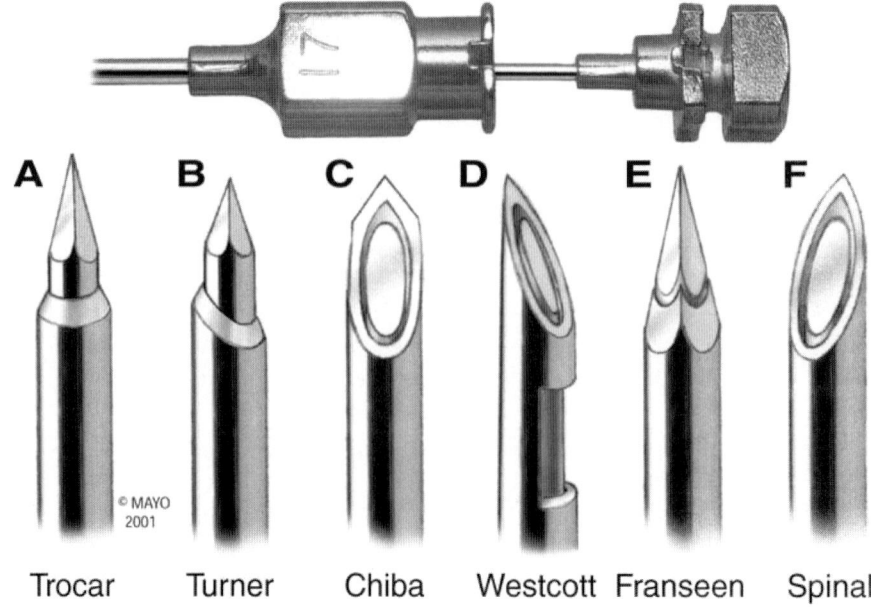

Fig. 1. Needle tips.

all-inclusive list nor a list of recommended equipment, but rather an example of various types of tools that can be used in a number of different procedures. Alterations in the composition of the set will be necessary according to the specific needs of the institutions where these procedures are performed.

Biopsy and Nonvascular Needles

FINE NEEDLE ASPIRATION BIOPSIES

These are performed with a higher gage needle attached to a syringe. Fine needle aspiration (FNA) biopsy is a percutaneous procedure that is typically accomplished with an 18–25g needle and may be performed under image guidance (i.e., CT or US). The area is first cleansed and then is numbed with local anesthetic. The needle is then placed into the tissue of interest, and a syringe is attached in order to aspirate the sample through the needle. Three to four samples are usually obtained. Before these samples are examined, the fluid may be placed in a centrifuge by the pathologist to separate the cells from the fluid. Masses within organs such as the liver, pancreas, lung, and thyroid have traditionally been amenable to FNA.

Chiba Needle

18–22 g, 6–20 cm length
  – Small-gage beveled tip (stylet and outer cannula) needle *(Fig. 1C)* usually used to gain initial access in nonvascular procedures; commonly used for procedures in the biliary and urinary tract.
  – These needles are available with US enhancement, which significantly increases the needle's visibility under US. The needle should initially be placed with the inner

stylet in place, as the enhancement on some needles is placed on the inner stylet (thereby allowing the outer cannula to remain smooth).

Franseen Needle

18–22 g, 6–20 cm length
  – Multibeveled tip (both stylet and outer cannula) needle *(Fig. 1E)* usually used for FNA biopsies. Particularly useful when the capillary technique is used to biopsy solid organs or nodules.

Spinal Needle

18–25 g, 5–15 cm in length
  – Beveled tip (both stylet and cannula) multipurpose needle *(Fig. 1F)* used for fluid aspiration, for injection of medications/contrast, and for biopsies.

Trocar Needle

18–21 g, 9–20 cm in length (also packaged in the Jeffrey Set)
  – Multibeveled inner stylet with flat, but tapered, outer cannula *(Fig. 1A)*. This needle may be used to gain access in nonvascular procedures or for biopsies. The Trocar needle is also often used for percutaneous abscess drainage (accepts a 0.035 inch guidewire).

Turner Needle

18–20 g, 9–20 cm in length
  – Similar in construction to the Trocar needle, with multibeveled inner stylet *(Fig. 1B)*, but the Turner needle has a slightly beveled outer cannula that is also tapered (circumferentially cutting edge). Its uses are similar to those of the Trocar needle.

Trucut, Surecut, Ata-cut, Auto-core, and Hepa-cut Needles

18–22 g, 5–20 cm in length

– These needles have attached syringes that may lock in place, thereby facilitating one-handed vacuum-assisted biopsies. These are available with an echogenic tip or needle shaft and have very sharp cutting edges. Aspiration/cutting needles provide the largest tissue core of any of the aspiration needles. Owing to the increased risk of pneumothorax and other lung complications, this needle is contraindicated for use in the lung.

Westcott Style Needle

20–22 g, 9–20 cm in length

– This needle has a beveled tip and a notched outer cannula (see Fig. 1D). The notch measures slightly over 2 mm and is located approx 3 mm from the tip of the needle. The slot creates a second cutting edge in addition to the needle tip. The notch allows aspiration of a larger amount of material.

Aspiration Needle

23–25 g, 4–5 cm in length

– Coated with an anticoagulant to minimize clotting within the inner core of the needle. Clear hub to facilitate immediate visualization of aspirate

Core Biopsy Needles

Core biopsy is performed by inserting a hollow needle through the skin and into the organ or mass to be investigated. The needle is carefully advanced into the tissue using image guidance. Core biopsy is often performed with the use of a spring-loaded device or gun (see Fig. 7) to assist in sampling and removing a small portion of the tissue of interest. The needle may be placed either by hand or with the assistance of a sampling device, and multiple insertions may be necessary to obtain an adequate sample. A coaxial technique can be used by which a smaller needle is inserted through a larger needle, which is left in the appropriate position while repeated biopsies are taken through the smaller needle. The core tissue samples are then sent to the pathology laboratory or presented to a pathologist present at the time of the procedure. This will allow the pathology lab to determine the adequacy of the sample and, possibly, to provide preliminary results.

Temno Needle

14–22 g, 6–20 cm in length

– Inner stylet with notch can be advanced into lesion before firing outer core over the inner stylet. This needle has an adjustable biopsy throw (1–2 cm) and an ultrasonographically echogenic tip. Available in coaxial biopsy sets.

Achieve Needle

14–20 g, 6–20 cm in length

– Inner stylet with notch can be advanced into the lesion before firing the outer core, or the needle can be placed on automatic mode for sequential firing. Available in coaxial biopsy sets. Echogenic marking is placed on the outer cannula.

AccuCore Needle

14–20 g, 9–15 cm in length

– Notched inner stylet with option of standard multibeveled point or sharper, multibeveled trocar point (available in 14 g, primarily intended for US-guided breast biopsies). Echogenic tip for US-guided biopsies. Inner stylet can be advanced into lesion before firing.

BioPince Biopsy Gun

18 g, 10–20 cm in length

– This biopsy gun delivers larger cylindrical core samples and is a single-action device. The throw length is adjustable, the stylet tip has a trocar style, and the needle tip functions as a pair of pincers. This biopsy gun has a very large (3.3-cm) stroke length, thereby allowing larger samples to be obtained than with comparable 18-g core biopsy needles. The needle tip, however, is not as easily controlled as in the devices that offer a controlled advance of the inner stylet.

Bard Biopsy Guns (Magnum and Monopty)

14–20 g, 10–25 cm in length

– Single-action biopsy gun that is available with different throw lengths.

Nonvascular Introducer Sets

Jeffrey Set

21-g needle, 15-cm length

– 0.018 inch Cope Mandril guidewire, 60-cm length
– Coaxial Catheter Introducer system

Stiffening cannula	20 g
Dilator	6.3 Fr, 20 cm length
Outer Sheath	8 Fr (OD) 17 cm length

Desilets-Hoffman Introducer Set

6.5 Fr

– Coaxial system
– Introducer dilator: inner diameter 0.038 inch
– Introducer sheath: Outer diameter 8.5 Fr, inner diameter 6.5 Fr or 0.086 inch

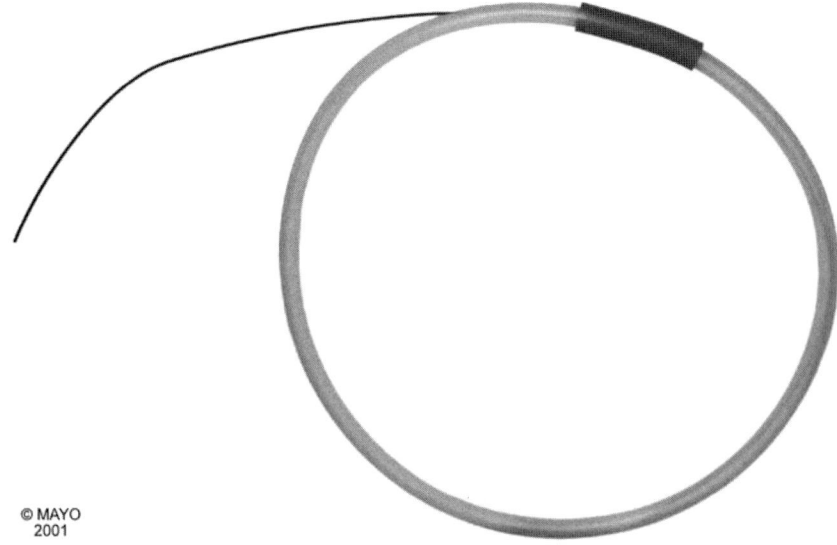

© MAYO
2001

Fig. 2. Bentson guidewire.

Guidewires

Guidewires are designed to allow the safe introduction and selective positioning of catheters. The typical guidewire consists of an outer spring and an inner core. The core can either be fixed or movable within the outer spring guide.

The ideal guidewire should be atraumatic, have a minimal friction surface, and be amenable to distal guidance from its proximal portion. Most guidewires are coated with Teflon and heparin to reduce friction and thrombogenecity. Some guidewires are coated with hydrophilic polymers, producing low coefficients of friction when wet. Generally, hydrophilic-polymer-coated guidewires are constructed of different materials (i.e., polymer plus nitinol wire core).

The guidewire size is expressed as diameter in inches. The diameter sizes can range from 0.010 to 0.045 inches. The standard length of a guidewire is 145 cm, with exchange lengths available up to 300 cm.

0.035-INCH DIAMETER

Bentson (Fig. 2)

Straight wire with floppy tip

145- and 200-cm lengths available

–A standard guidewire with a 15-cm flexible distal tip.

Terumo Glidewire (Fig. 3)

Angled and J-shaped distal tip

145 cm length

–Hydrophilic-coated material improves tracking and negotiation through narrow channels.

–Guidewire of choice for initial crossing of a distal common bile duct obstruction. If the wire is placed

through a beveled access needle and withdrawn, segments of the wire may be sheared off.

Amplatz Stiff/Extra Stiff/Super Stiff (Fig. 4)

Straight tip

145 cm length; Super Stiff available in 210 and 260 cm lengths *(Fig. 4)*

–Stiff shaft with gradual transition to a flexible tip. Traditionally, but not exclusively, used in nonvascular procedures. A different inner core adds stiffness to the Extra- and Superstiff wires. The stiffest wires are especially useful for biliary drainage placements or tube changes.

0.018-INCH DIAMETER

Torq-Flex

Straight tip

60 and 200 cm lengths

–Stiff shaft wire with an 8-cm distal stainless steel spring coil tip. A short Torq-Flex wire is packaged in the micropuncture set (*see* Chapter 4).

Cope Mandril

Straight tip

60 cm length

–Stainless steel guidewire that is very stiff and has a platinum spring coil tip. The shaft of the guidewire is comparable to a 0.035-inch guidewire. The Cope-Mandril guidewire is packaged in the Jeffrey Set and is used for many nonvascular interventions such as biliary drainage and nephrostomy tube placement.

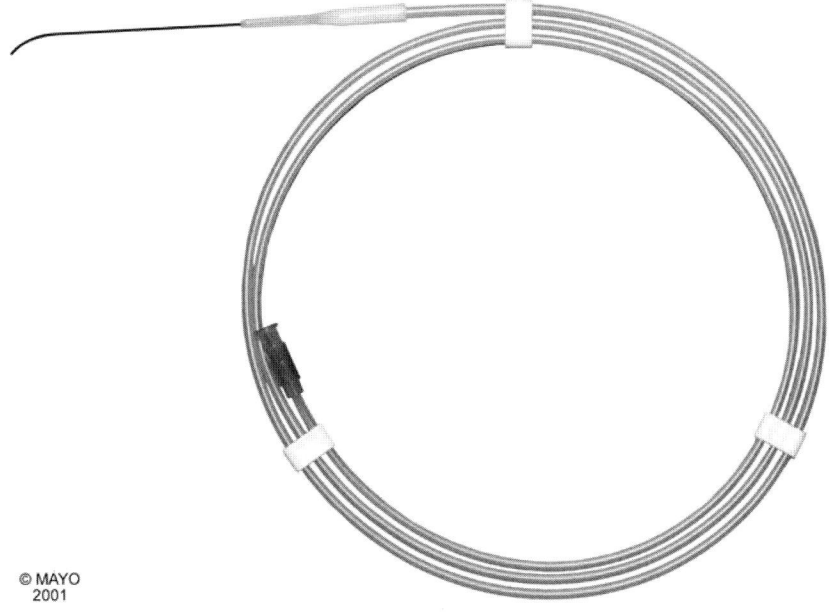

© MAYO
2001

Fig. 3. Terumo glidewire (angled).

Nonvascular Catheters

Percuflex Biliary Drainage Catheter

8.0–14 Fr

35 cm length

– Percuflex catheters have a hydrophilic coating that reduces friction and buckling during advancement through the liver or tight strictures. The catheter is softer and more comfortable for the patient than a ring catheter. The system has a locking mechanism that may retain the pigtail shape in the duodenum

Ring Biliary Drainage Catheter

8.3 Fr; 32, 41, or 63 sideholes

55 cm length

– Polyethylene catheter with multiple sideholes for biliary drainage. Ring catheter material is stiffer than the Percuflex.

Heyer-Schulte Catheter

12–24 Fr

Custom-fit length

– Silicone material with multiple sideholes placed for long-term biliary drainage. This catheter is made from softer and more pliable material and has a larger lumen and sideholes.

Van Andel Catheter

5–12 Fr

Variable length

– This is a Teflon catheter with a tapered tip that is used for advancement of other catheters (i.e., Heyer-Schulte catheter) or to predilate a tract in preparation for additional interventions.

Mueller Catheter

8.3 Fr with 16 sideholes

50 cm length

– Straight polyethylene catheter with multiple distal sideholes. Often used if crossing the biliary obstruction is unsuccessful. The Mueller catheter is positioned above the obstruction and opened to external drainage. After the biliary ducts are decompressed, an additional attempt can be made to cross the obstruction. This catheter may also be used for over-the-wire cholangiogram or nephrostogram. In combination with the Tuohy-Bourst (Y-adapter), contrast is injected while maintaining access with the guidewire.

Kaufman Catheter

8 Fr with 41 sideholes

50cm length

– Stiff Teflon catheter used to cross high-grade biliary or urinary strictures.

APD (All Purpose Drainage) Catheter

8 and 10 Fr

25 cm length

– Commonly used for percutaneous abscess drainage.

Vansonnenberg Chest Drainage Catheter

12 and 14 Fr

25 cm length

– Single-lumen catheter for percutaneous abscess drainage.

Vansonnenberg Sump Catheter

12–16 Fr

30 cm length

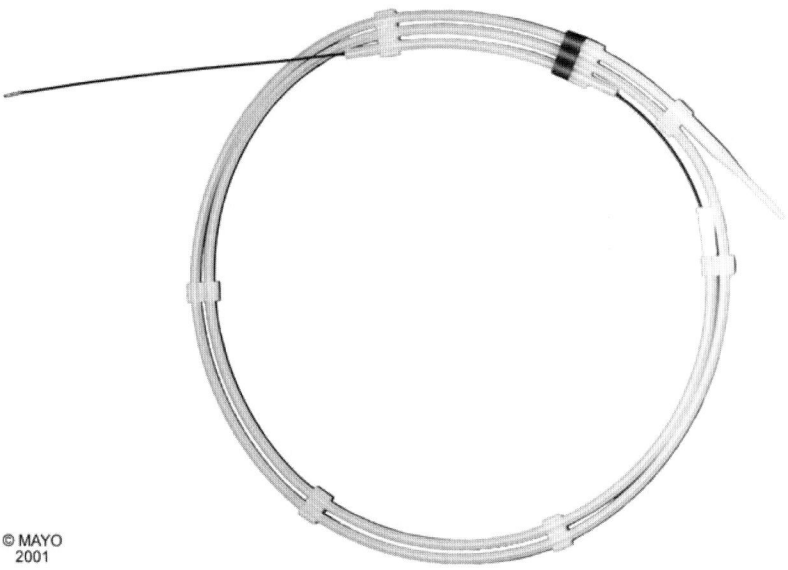

© MAYO
2001

Fig. 4. Amplatz Super Stiff guidewire.

–A dual-lumen catheter with two inner channels. Drainage occurs through the larger lumen. The smaller lumen is designed to allow air to enter the cavity (through a Millipore filter), creating a venting effect.

Straight Drainage Catheter

8–14 Fr

Length varies

–Multiusage drainage catheter; additional sideholes may be added.

Percuflex Nephrostomy Catheter

8–16 Fr

25 cm in length

–Hydrophilic coated catheter to ease advancement and prevent buckling. Locking mechanism is available on the nephrostomy catheter.

Hopkins Percutaneous Catheter

8–14 Fr

Length varies

–Pigtail with six sideholes, used for nephrostomy conversion to ureteral stent. Additional sideholes are added depending on the length between the kidney and bladder.

Miscellaneous Abdominal Interventions

The etiology of various abdominal fluid collections is important for planning an approach for intervention and treatment. Regardless of the modality used in diagnosis, the radiologist must carefully analyze all objective data before draining the fluid collection. Contraindications to performing percutaneous drainage must be carefully examined and addressed, and therapy should begin as soon as is clinically feasible to prevent delay or deterioration in the patient's clinical condition.

CONTRAINDICATIONS, LABORATORY VALUES, AND PREPROCEDURE THERAPY

For patients undergoing various nonvascular interventional procedures, the prothrombin time/partial thrombo-plastin time (PT/PTT) and platelet count may be checked. For patients with no history of a bleeding disorder and no other complicating factors, the procedure can be done without preprocedure lab values according to the discretion of the treating physician.

If the coagulation factors are significantly abnormal, such as a PT greater than 1.5 times the normal range or an INR (international normalized ratio) time greater than 1.5 times the top normal range, these factors should be corrected before performing the procedure (except in absolute emergencies). The platelet count should be greater than 50,000, and other coagulation parameters should be within normal limits. If the platelet count is less than 50,000, a platelet transfusion should be considered before the procedure.

For procedures with potential for bacterial contamination, antibiotics should be administered. The antibiotic should be selected based on the results from prior cultures or on the type of bacteria likely to be encountered. If this information is unknown or unavailable, a wide-spectrum antibiotic should be considered.

DRAINAGE OF FLUID COLLECTIONS

Postoperative Abscesses

Despite advances in surgical care and perioperative antibiotic regimens, postoperative abdominal abscesses continue to be a problem. Cross-sectional imaging allows prompt and accurate diagnosis of postoperative abscesses and can guide percutaneous drainage procedures.

The timing of imaging studies in the postoperative period is important. Intraabdominal fluid resulting from intraoperative irrigation, inflammatory changes, and edema may decrease the sensitivity for detecting early abscess formation. The eighth postoperative day is a commonly accepted time to perform cross-sectional imaging in patients with symptoms suggesting a postoperative infection. This postoperative time interval allows for reabsorption of nonsuppurative fluid collections and resolution of swelling in otherwise normal tissue. When the presence of a postoperative infection is uncertain, percutaneous aspiration of a fluid sample can provide culture and sensitivity information as well as more immediate results from a Gram stain.

In the presence of infection, percutaneous drainage can either be used as a temporizing measure or for obviating the need for surgical intervention altogether. Limitations to percutaneous drainage, however, do exist and include surgical anastomotic dehiscence, the presence of multiple loculations within an abscess, excessive cellular debris, or an inadequate percutaneous drainage route. All these potential limitations may limit or prevent the successful percutaneous drainage of a postoperative fluid collection.

Any drainage catheter that is placed for the purpose of abscess drainage should be left in place until there is no longer any clinical or imaging evidence of infection. Premature removal of the drainage catheter may predispose to recurrence of the abscess and could necessitate a second drainage procedure (percutaneous or surgical).

Appendiceal Abscesses

Appendicitis remains one of the most commonly encountered acute illnesses that frequently require surgery. Although the diagnosis has been typically based on physical examination findings and clinical data, recent advances in management of acute appendicitis have focused on prompt preoperative imaging evaluation in an attempt to avoid unnecessary laparotomies. US and CT have provided valuable additional information that will allow the treating physician the opportunity to elect for image-guided intervention if an appendiceal perforation and abscess are present.

Diverticular Disease

US and CT have made the accurate diagnosis and anatomic definition of acute diverticulitis possible. Current standard management depends on accurate diagnosis, the condition of the patient, and the extent of extracolonic involvement. Over the past few years, image-guided intervention has complemented traditional surgical treatments in the definitive management of patients with diverticulitis.

The treatment of diverticulitis is dependent on the severity of the disease. Traditionally multistage surgical procedures were used to treat patients with more severe diverticular disease including abscesses and fecal peritonitis from diverticular rupture. By draining peridiverticular abscesses, percutaneous fluid drainages may obviate or decrease the need for multiple abdominal surgeries.

Pancreatic Disease

Cholelithiasis and alcoholism account for the most cases of pancreatitis seen in the United States. Contrast-enhanced CT has become the imaging modality of choice and allows accurate estimations of the size, location, and extent of inflammatory change. This information is extremely important if aspiration is considered because of superimposed infection or the presence of a very large pancreatic pseudocyst. Fluid collections >7-cm in diameter are more likely to require intervention, especially if they are caused by alcohol-induced pancreatitis. Approximately half of the acute fluid collections resolve spontaneously, and drainage procedures are not indicated until they mature into pseudocysts or become infected.

Pancreatic necrosis involves injury to the acinar, islet, and ductal cells and results in extensive fat necrosis and focal regions of nonviable pancreatic tissue. Contrast-enhanced spiral CT will demonstrate nonenhancing pancreatic parenchyma (<50 Hounsfield units [HU] of enhancement in a more than 3-cm area of the pancreatic parenchyma or in >30% of the gland). When pancreatic necrosis is present, the secondary bacterial infection rate can be as high as 40–60%. In the presence of necrotic or severe pancreatitis, it is important to differentiate between fluid and nonliquid inflammatory change, as the latter cannot be aspirated despite the use of a large-gage needle.

Percutaneous drainage has been suggested either as a strategy for primary therapy or as a temporizing measure in critically ill patients before surgical intervention. Image-guided therapy is now an important adjunct to current management techniques in treating patients with pancreatic pseudocysts. Percutaneous drainage must be considered in patients whom are poor surgical candidates but have persistent symptoms related to their pseudocysts.

The primary disadvantages of percutaneous drainage of peripancreatic fluid collections include the risk of developing an external pancreatic fistula and the significant commitment to tube management once the initial drainage tube is placed. Before placing a drainage catheter, one must consider the possibility that the tube (or a series of tubes) may remain in place for many weeks.

Preprocedure Management

Abdominal and retroperitoneal interventions are numerous and varied according to the specific clinical indication. Each patient, must be evaluated however, before an invasive procedure. A consultation for written evaluation should be documented in the patients' chart, and informed consent should be obtained before performing the procedure. Results of the consultation should be discussed with the managing clinical team when appropriate. A clinical care plan should be developed, and an attempt should be made to estimate the potential problems that could either delay the procedure or result from the procedure itself. Appropriate notification of preprocedural problems should be given to avoid having the patient sent to the Radiology Department prematurely.

A consultation should include the following information:

- Service performing procedure, date, time, patients name, referring physician
- History of the present illness
- Past medical and surgical history
- Medications
- Allergies (including reactions to iodinated contrast)
- Diagnostic test results (including those from outside institutions)
- Directed physical exam
  - Vital signs
  - Heart, lung, abdomen, and other examination data pertinent to the impending procedure
- Pertinent laboratory data (*see* Contraindications, Laboratory Values, and Preprocedure Therapy section above)
- Brief results of previous imaging studies
- Assessment of patient
- Clinical care plan
- Signature.

Preprocedure Orders

These orders, when necessary, usually include instructions for diet, intravenous fluids, antibiotics, and any necessary preprocedure lab work. Occasionally, special situations will arise that should be addressed in the preprocedure orders. Some of these situations are described below.

Diet

Patients undergoing general anesthesia must be NPO after midnight the night before the procedure and patients receiving conscious sedation should be on a clear liquid diet for 8–12 h before the procedure. Diabetic patients will require extra preprocedural attention and should reduce their insulin dosage the morning of the procedure. Diabetic patients on an oral hypoglycemic medication should hold their morning dose on the day of their intervention.

Antibiotics

The use of antibiotics before some invasive procedures reduces the rate of postprocedure infection. The most common of these clinical situations include biliary and urinary tract manipulations.

Intravenous Fluids

Many patients will require venous access and/or iv fluids before entering the procedure room. Common fluid orders include:

- D-5-W NS @ KVO (keep vessel open) approx 20–30 mL/h
- NS @ KVO or 60–70 mL/h for diabetic patients
- IV with Heplock for patients on chronic hemodialysis and other patients with fluid restrictions

Anticoagulated Patients

Patients on Coumadin® should have their medication stopped for at least 5 days. Patients on heparin should have it stopped 2–4 h before the procedure. The PT/PTT should be rechecked for patients taking Coumadin.

Patients with a History of Contrast Reaction

Document the severity of the reaction (i.e., hives, rash, laryngeal edema, and so on), and administer one of the premedication protocols:

- Prednisone 40 mg PO: two doses, one 12–18 h before the exam and one 2 h before exam, *or*
- Three doses: 24, 12, and 2 h before exam, *or*
- Solu-Corteif® 100 mg iv 12 hours and 2 h before the exam, *and*
- Benadryl® 50 mg PO 1 h before the exam is given in addition to the corticosteroids
- An H-2 blocker such as Pepcid®, 20 mg iv can also be given before the procedure.

Procedures

The various invasive image-guided procedures are too numerous and complex to be addressed in a single section, chapter, or comprehensive manual. In addition to drainages of fluid collections common nonvascular invasive procedures include abdominal/retroperitoneal biopsies, lung biopsies (described in Section 2), and percutaneous nephrostomy tube placement.

When using an imaging modality that produces ionizing radiation (i.e., fluoroscopy, CT), always wear lead apron protection and a radiation dosimetry badge. Lead-based thyroid and eye protection is also recommended when ionizing radiation is used. Universal precautions should always be observed to protect against the unintended exposure to blood and body fluids. The appropriate size of sterile gloves can allow more unencumbered hand movement and may facilitate optimal manual dexterity. Double gloving is always recommended, as there is a continual risk of exposure to such blood-borne pathogens as HIV and hepatitis C.

Before preparing for the procedure, always introduce yourself to the patient and be available to answer any last minute questions he or she may have. After the patients' questions have been answered and concerns addressed, the physician performing the procedure and any direct assistants should start by scrubbing their hands.

The scrub protocol is variable. For sterile procedures such as an indwelling tunneled catheter placement or in patients who are immunosuppressed, a complete surgical scrub is necessary. For most other procedures, a light scrub with sterile gloves and a gown will suffice.

The procedure tray and table should be prepared sometime before scrubbing or directly before the procedure. The patient will need to be prepped by using either an iodine-based solution (i.e., Betadine®) or, in patients with an allergy or sensitivity to Betadine, a non-iodine-based solution such as Hibiclens® (chlorhexidine gluconate and isopropyl alcohol). The degree of antibacterial activity of the skin preparation solution is related to contact time with the skin. The antibacterial solution, therefore, should be placed as early in the patient preparation process as possible.

In addition to the local anesthetic, iv medications given as part of a conscious sedation protocol provide an enormous benefit in terms of facilitating patient comfort. Two of the most commonly used medications are midazolam (Versed®) and Fentanyl®. A standard dose is 1 mg of midazolam and 50 µg of Fentanyl. Common jargon indicating a single administration of the above amounts of these medications is a "one and one."

Patient monitoring during conscious sedation is a necessity. Monitoring and support devices include electrocardiography (ECG), pulse oximeter, and blood pressure. The patient may also be given supplemental oxygen via nasal cannula or facemask. (Care must be taken not to suppress the drive to breathe in patients with chronic obstructive pulmonary disease.)

Sample Procedure

PERCUTANEOUS NEPHROSTOMY

This procedure is typically done to divert the flow of urine, usually in an attempt to bypass an obstruction. Although this procedure is commonly performed, major complications such as sepsis, hemorrhage, and kidney injury can occur in as many as 5% of patients even when it is performed by experienced physicians.

The basic steps in performing a percutaneous nephrostomy tube (PNT) placement include:

1. Patient preparation
2. Collecting system visualization
3. Puncture site selection
4. Collecting system puncture
5. Tract dilation
6. Catheter insertion and fixation
7. Patient follow-up

Preprocedural preparation should be accomplished as described above including explaining the procedure, obtaining informed consent, and ordering the appropriate laboratory tests. Any coagulopathy should be corrected before the procedure; the patient's INR should not exceed 1.5, and their platelet count should be a minimum of 50,000. To minimize the risk of sepsis, antibiotics should be given before the procedure. Broad-spectrum antibiotic coverage such as ampicillin (2 g given iv every 6 h) or gentamycin (1.5 mg/kg given iv every 8 h) should provide adequate prophylaxis. If an oral regimen is desired, ciprofloxacin can be given (500 mg po every 12 h). Antibiotics should be given approximately 1 h before the procedure and can be discontinued after placement of the PNT if there are no clinical signs of infection.

Collecting system visualization, puncture site selection, and puncture selection should be done very carefully to minimize the risk of hemorrhage. The posterolateral kidney is a relatively avascular portion called the Brodel bloodless line of incision and an ideal approach is to puncture the end of a posterior calyx in this region (see Fig. 5). The posterior calyces are usually oriented so that their long axes point through the avascular zone of the kidney. Therefore, visualization of the appropriate calyx for puncture is helpful to minimize hemorrhagic complications.

The collecting system can be visualized by using multiple techniques including injecting iv contrast, retrograde injection of contrast via an indwelling ureteral catheter, or injecting contrast antegrade though a small needle in an attempt to opacify the renal pelvis or a posterior calyx. Sonographic, CT, or fluoroscopic guidance can all be used in the placement of a PNT. A nephrostomy tube can be placed with sonography alone or in combination with fluoroscopic guidance. In some patients in whom limiting the amount of ionizing radiation is important (i.e., pregnant patients), sonography should be used to minimize the radiation dose.

The procedure is performed with the patient in a prone position. A posterior calyx is located using the modality of choice, and the initial puncture is made with a 22-g needle. (The risk of a clinically important hemorrhage is negligible when a 22-g needle is used for the initial renal puncture.) If necessary, a blind puncture can be performed just lateral to the vertebral transverse process at the L1-L2 level. When executing a blind puncture, the needle is passed directly vertical to the collecting system during interrupted breathing. As the needle is withdrawn, urine is aspirated and a small amount is retained for culture. A small volume of contrast is then injected through the needle using fluoroscopic monitoring to confirm the position of the needle within the collecting system. A small volume of air (5–10 mL) can also be injected into the collecting system to define the posterior calyces better. Air should be injected carefully and only after the intrapelvocalyceal location of the needle tip is confirmed. Injection of air into a vessel can cause air embolization. With the patient prone, the room air rises into the posterior calyces, thereby making them conspicuous.

In difficult cases, US or CT can be used during renal entry to visualize orientation of the calyces better. Image guidance can be especially helpful in patients with an unusual body habitus such as those individuals with severe scoliosis, hepatosplenomegaly, or ectopic kidney position.

During the injection of iodinated contrast and/or air, it is important to avoid overdistention of the intrarenal collecting system. This can force a backflow of infected urine into the venous system, thereby significantly increasing the risk of septicemia. Overdistention can be avoided by aspirating as much or more volume than is injected.

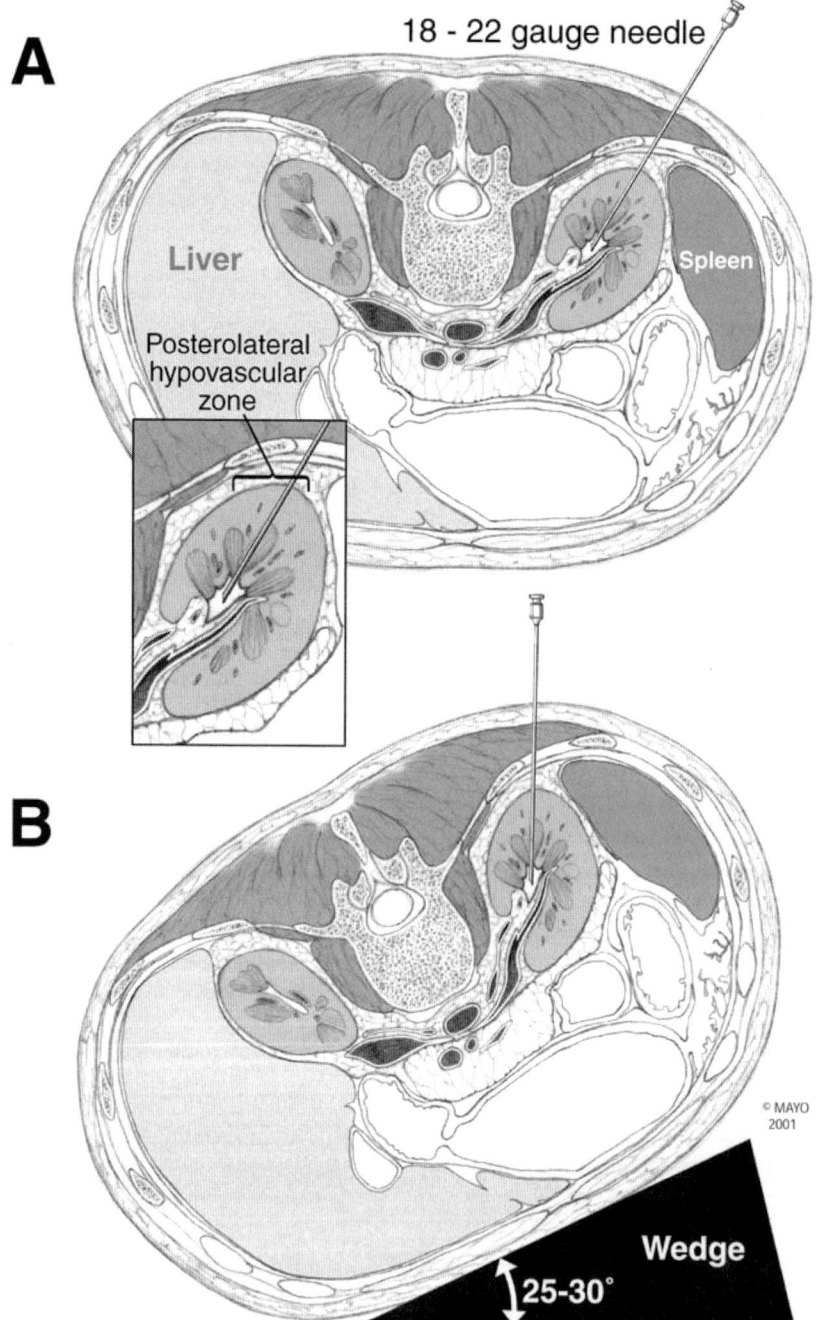

Fig. 5. Percutaneous nephrostomy tube placement.

(A) Angled needle approach: the patient is placed prone, and the needle is angled sufficiently at allow the puncture of a posterior calyx through the posterolateral hypovascular zone (Brodel's bloodless line of incision.

(B) Patient angled approach: a positioning wedge is placed under the patient to produce a 25–30-degree anterior oblique position. The needle can then be directed vertically into a posterior calyx through the hypovascular zone.

 The needle angled technique has the advantage of requiring less patient positioning, and the patient angled approach has the advantage that the needle can be directed vertically.

 Once the collecting system has been visualized, a calyx should be selected in which to create a percutaneous nephrostomy tract by means of a second needle puncture with image guidance. Site selection depends on renal position and the antic- ipated need for future interventions. If an antegrade advance- ment of the ureteral stent is anticipated, a superior pole calyx makes this advancement much easier than a lower pole calyx. In general, when additional ureteral manipulations are anticipated, a middle to upper pole calyx should be selected for the initial PNT placement location. Additionally, renal position should also be considered and the puncture point should ideally be below the 12th rib, thereby avoiding transpleural nephrostomy tracts. Puncture of the kidney between the 11th and 12th ribs, is frequently necessary, but puncture above the 11th rib should be avoided, as transpleural passage is likely at this level.

Single-wall calyceal punctures are preferable to avoid injury to larger renal vessels and should be used to decrease the likelihood of a clinically significant hemorrhage. If one of the larger vessels ventral to the renal pelvis is injured by passing through both walls of the renal pelvis, the bleeding will not be stopped by nephrostomy tube insertion. Bleeding caused by a dorsal vessel injury during a single wall puncture, however, should be occluded by the subsequent placement of the nephrostomy tube.

For calyceal puncture, as for all abscess or fluid collection aspirations where the placement of a drainage catheter is anticipated, an 18-g needle should be used. This needle size will accept a 0.035-inch guidewire and also provides additional stiffness that allows very little needle bending or misdirection. Alternatively, the selected calyx can be punctured with a smaller 22-g needle that will accept a 0.018-inch guidewire. A coaxial dilator can be advanced over the wire and the tract then dilated. Subsequently, the smaller guidewire can be replaced with a 0.035-inch wire for further manipulation.

As mentioned previously, calyceal puncture should be made posterolaterally at an angle 20–30 degrees from vertical. This should ensure puncture of the renal parenchyma through the relatively avascular region. Before puncture, the needle pathway should be examined for intervening structures (i.e., colon) that may be between the skin and the calyceal target. Approximately 5% of patients will have a retrorenal position of their colon when lying prone. The retrorenal colon, when present, is usually gas-filled and easy to identify. The colon must be avoided when placing a PNT.

Once the calyx has been punctured and a stable wire has been placed, a catheter should be advanced over the guidewire. Contrast material should always be injected before catheter placement to confirm an intracollecting system position before dilating the tube tract. Care must be taken to maintain percutaneous access to the intrarenal collecting system once initial access is established. Percutaneous puncture of an obstructed system increases the risk of bacteremia and sepsis, and urinary tract manipulations should be kept to a minimum in these patients.

For percutaneous urinary drainage, 8- or 10-Fr nephrostomy catheters are standard. If the urine is visibly infected or contains a substantial amount of debris, a 10-Fr or larger catheter is often used to provide adequate drainage of viscous fluid that may be present. When long-term drainage is needed, self-retaining nephrostomy catheters should be used to minimize the risk of dislodging the catheter.

In hospitalized patients, routine follow-up of the patients should be performed on a daily basis for the first few days to ensure adequate urine output, decreasing hematuria, and a decrease in the amount of discomfort at the PNT insertion site. Lack of resolution or persistence of symptoms suggest a complication such as tube occlusion, vascular injury, or tube malposition. Prompt identification of any complications will facilitate the appropriate treatment and increase the chances of successful resolution of any untoward events.

Despite the most cautious approach, complications occasionally occur during the placement of a PNT. Following these guidelines will minimize the patient's risk and will keep the complication rate to a minimum. Most of the more common complications associated with PNT placement (i.e., colonic puncture, renal vascular injury, and transpleural tube placement) are treated nonsurgically; with careful technique, more severe complications such as severe sepsis and extensive hemorrhage can be avoided in nearly all patients.

Postprocedure Management

The goal of postprocedure management is to ensure the patient's safety and stable recovery while facilitating an expeditious discharge from the department. In cases requiring immediate postprocedure care, the primary care team should be contacted directly after or toward the end of the procedure.

FUTURE INDWELLING CATHETERS AND/OR TUBES TO THE SKIN

Indwelling tubes such as biliary, nephrostomy, and abscess drainage tubes should be secured at the skin surface. Most indwelling tubes can be secured by using a nonabsorbable microfilament suture (either 2-0 or 3-0 nylon). These sutures should be removed after two weeks. Silk may be used to mark the tubes at the skin surface but should not be used to suture the tube to the skin, given the inflammatory reaction associated with the subcutaneous placement of the silk. Those individuals not facile with tying surgical knots may want to review and practice the two-hand technique for surgical ties.

WRITE A POSTPROCEDURE NOTE IN THE CHART

Subject headings include:

–Preprocedure diagnosis

–Postprocedure diagnosis

–Procedure

–Physicians

–Contrast

–Medications

–Complications

–Findings

–Interpretation/conclusions

–Disposition

WRITE POSTPROCEDURE ORDERS FOR THE PATIENT

Generally, postoperative procedure orders include vitals, pulse, wound checks, diet, pain management, tube drainage management, lab work, and antibiotic coverage. Record a time, date, and signature for all orders and progress notes. A physician must also sign the order sheet and the nurse's flow sheet for conscious sedation. Some patients are held in the recovery room for evaluation and management. The physician, along with the personnel in the recovery room, will determine if, how, and how long the patient is monitored. There are usually specific protocols for monitoring and criteria for discharge. These will vary from institution to institution, and knowledge of these policies is important to facilitate the appropriate recovery room care and patient transfer.

An example of postprocedure orders for a percutaneous biliary tube placement is as follows:

- Bed rest 1–6 h (shorter if outpatient)
- Monitor vital signs (1–6 h)
  - Q 15 min × 4
  - Q 30 min × 4
  - Q 1 h × 3
- Resume diet/fluids as tolerated
- Continue iv

- Monitor bile output every shift and record
- Replace bile every shift mL for mL with lactated Ringer's solution
- Hydroxycodone 1–2 tablets PO or meperidine 50–75mg IM q 3–4 h prn pain
- Continue antibiotic coverage for 2–4 doses (24 h), except for gentamycin, which is given as a single, preprocedural dose
- Bile sample sent to lab for culture and sensitivity.

PRINT OR STORE SELECTED FILMS

Select the images that best represent and/or demonstrate the findings of a case. The extra images from the case can either be stored electronically or placed in a secondary jacket.

DICTATE THE CASE

Cases should optimally be dictated in very close proximity to the conclusion of the procedure, and the transcribed report should be finalized within 24 h. If necessary for billing purposes, the physician should dictate exactly what procedures were done.

2 LUNG BIOPSY

Needle aspiration and biopsy of intrathoracic pathology has been one of the most common imaging-guided procedures for many years. Despite this prior experience, transthoracic biopsy continues to be challenging and should be limited to cases with an identifiable indication and those that are technically feasible. Complication and specimen retrieval rates, even among experienced personnel, vary widely. A unified approach to transthoracic biopsy that will maximize the chances of obtaining a specimen while minimizing the potential complications is therefore necessary if one is to perform this procedure successfully.

Biopsy Equipment

Modality Choice

Although CT guidance offers many advantages in percutaneous transthoracic lung biopsy in a patient with relatively normal lung parenchyma and a lesion that is well visualized in two projections on plain film radiography, fluoroscopic guidance offers some advantages. Generally fluoroscopic biopsies are faster, and the room costs are lower. Additionally, the lesion can be viewed in real time, and the ribs can be avoided more easily than when working under CT guidance. The needle can also be advanced under direct visualization using a surgical clamp, and the lung lesion may be "shaken," thereby confirming appropriate positioning of the needle. If patients are cooperative and if the lung parenchyma is relatively normal, even small lesions that are visible under fluoroscopy may be biopsied fairly quickly and with a high degree of accuracy.

In spite of the longer procedure duration, CT offers several important advantages. CT is the safest and most accurate method of biopsying central lesions and lesions adjacent to or involving the hila and mediastinal structures. The cross-sectional view also allows anatomic hazards such as bullae/blebs, large vessels, and the pulmonary fissures to be avoided. Occasionally CT can identify lesions that have benign characteristics, obviating the need for biopsy, and can also identify portions of necrotic tumors that are more likely to contain viable tissue that will be representative of the lesion.

Needle Choice

As recently as the mid-1990s, survey data have shown that most lung biopsies in the United States were being performed using the single-needle technique. Despite its widespread use, this technique has few advantages over a coaxial technique that involves inserting a needle through the cannula of a slightly larger needle and into the pulmonary lesion *(Fig. 6)*. The coaxial technique has the primary advantage of limiting the number of pleural punctures, thereby decreasing the risk of the most common complication of lung biopsy, a pneumothorax.

Each pleural puncture site has the potential to cause an air leak, and each site has a unique and reproducible pressure above which an air leak will occur. With a coaxial technique, a number of samples can be obtained through the outer needle without introducing other needles and without making additional punctures of the pleural surfaces. With most needles, the depth of the sampling process can be adjusted, and the outer needle is usually rigid enough to allow substantial directional torque to be applied without bending it. The outer needle usually prevents air leakage and can also be used to take a larger

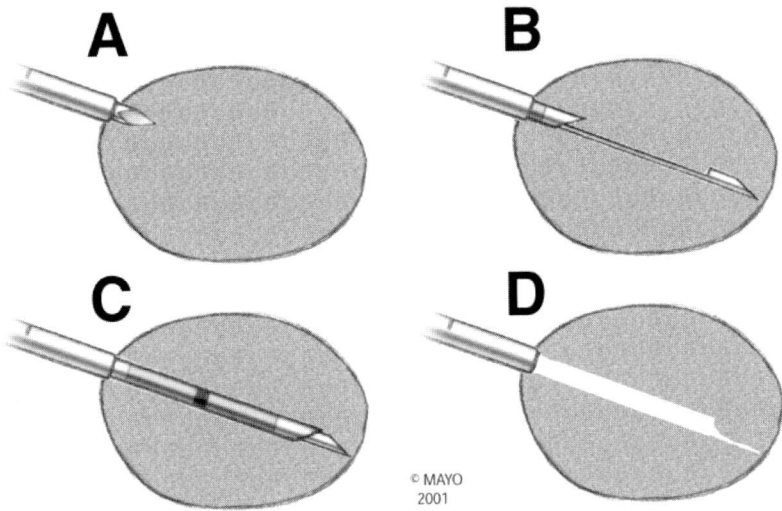

Fig. 6. Coaxial technique.

(A) The outer needle is placed into the proximal portion of the lesion, and the inner stylet is then removed.
(B) The biopsy needle is advanced into the lesion. When a dual-action core biopsy needle (shown) is used, the inner needle is advanced into the lesion.
(C) The biopsy is obtained (via the capillary technique with fine needle aspiration biopsies or by firing the core biopsy device shown).
(D) The tissue is obtained, and the cannula of the outer needle is left in place. The inner stylet of the needle is reinserted between biopsies.

gage sample through the lesion itself. At the conclusion of the procedure, the outer needle may be used to deliver a blood patch (discussed below). Regardless of the position of the pulmonary lesion, care must be taken to ensure that the outer cannula of the coaxial system is inside the pleural surfaces, as multiple pleural punctures resulting from an outer cannula placed outside the parietal pleura can dramatically increase the chance of a pneumothorax.

In certain cases the use of a single needle would be advantageous. When a biopsy of a large nonnecrotic mass is performed, the single-needle technique can usually obtain an adequate sample and is less expensive than the coaxial system. When normal intrathoracic structures (i.e., the superior vena cava [SVC]) must be transgressed in order to give access to the site of interest, smaller gage needles are less traumatic and may decrease complication rates. In hemorrhagic lesions, the thinner single needle is also preferred in order to decrease the likelihood of significant pulmonary hemorrhage.

Needle Type

The two basic needle types used for lung biopsy are needles for FNA and core biopsy needles. After the initial CT scan is obtained and before a biopsy is performed, the physician should decide whether the lesion is likely to represent a neoplasm. If malignancy is suspected, a FNA should be obtained before attempts at core biopsy. Core biopsy needles slightly increase the risk of complications such as hemorrhage and air embolism but improve the accuracy of diagnosis in benign disease processes and certain types of lymphoma. Although core biopsy devices may be used on most lung lesions, they should ideally

be reserved for situations in which a lesion other than a neoplasm is biopsied or when more material is needed to make a definitive diagnosis.

Core biopsy needles should be, light, compact, and easy to use and should reliably produce a core biopsy specimen that is adequate for histologic evaluation. Modern coaxial models (Fig. 7) come in a variety of lengths and provide an outer needle to use as a guide along with an inner needle that has an adjustable throw length. The adjustable throw length is an important option, as the transgression of normal lung tissue should be kept to a minimum.

Few studies have compared the safety and complication rates of the various needle types used for lung biopsies. A variety of needle tips are available, including a standard point, trocar point, Franseen tip, single/triple/rounded bevel, needle point, and beveled needle with a slotted outer cannula. All such needles are probably acceptable, but needles that have any feature predisposing toward a linear pleural tear should be avoided. Generally smaller gage needles (18 g or smaller) should be used, as large-gage needles are considered to place the patient at increased risk of hemorrhage and pneumothorax.

Preparation

In preparing for a lung biopsy, the case should be examined to determine that the procedure can be done without undue risk to the patient and that the results will be a crucial informational component in the patient's plan for treatment. Other considerations will include the likelihood of successfully obtaining a diagnostic specimen and any patient risk factors that could increase the risk of procedural complications.

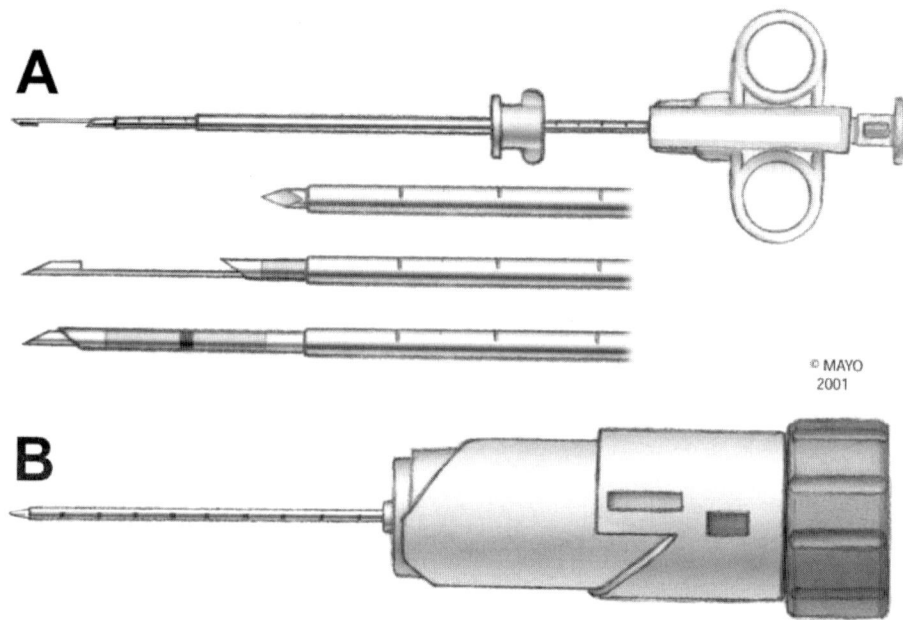

© MAYO
2001

Fig. 7. Core biopsy devices.

(A) Dual-action core biopsy needle. This needle is usually packed with the outer guiding needle and is placed through the outer cannula after the inner stylet of the outer guiding needle has been removed (shown). The inner needle can be advanced into the lesion before firing the biopsy device. Once the biopsy device is triggered, the outer cannula of the core biopsy needle slides quickly over the inner needle, thereby obtaining tissue within the notch in the inner needle.

(B) Single-action core biopsy gun. This device operates in an analogous way to the dual-action needle but does not allow for advancement of the inner needle into the lesion before obtaining the biopsy. The biopsy is obtained after the biopsy device is triggered.

Review of the patient's CT scan, chest X-ray, and medical history is crucial; laboratory data should also be reviewed as part of the preprocedure planning. Such obstacles as superficial blebs or vascular structures can be noted and a plan constructed to avoid them. The risk of pneumothorax is also significantly increased in the presence of emphysema, obstructive lung disease, and AIDS. In all these patients, as well as in patients with only one lung (or with a contiguous pleural space), it is advisable to prepare the skin site for insertion of a thoracostomy tube and to have the appropriate equipment for tube insertion ready for immediate use.

When an increased risk of pulmonary hemorrhage is perceived, bronchoscopic backup should be available in order to tamponade a bleeding site if necessary. Intubation should generally be avoided in patients with pulmonary hemorrhage but, when necessary, is optimally performed with a double-lumen tube. Personnel experience in double-lumen intubation should be available as part of a prudent approach to lung biopsy.

All patients should have various vital functions monitored during the exam with a cardiac monitor, pulse oximetry, and blood pressure cuff. All patients should have iv access, as conscious sedation is very helpful in patients undergoing lung biopsy, and iv access is occasionally needed to deliver medications (i.e., atropine in patients with severe vasovagal responses) and intravascular volume in those patients with significant bleeding or hypotension. Other supplemental equip-

ment should be readily available including oxygen, an oral airway, a ventilation bag and mask, and suction equipment. In addition to this preparation, equipment used to aspirate a pneumothorax also needs to be available and identified before the procedure. This includes small-bore chest tubes, an intravenous catheter or spinal needle, suction device (wall- or self-contained), and the appropriate tubing.

Before performing a transthoracic biopsy, all physicians must be familiar with the appropriate treatments for a vasovagal reaction, significant hemoptysis, and air embolism and should be certified in basic and advanced cardiac life support. A resuscitation cart should be immediately available, either in the biopsy suite itself or nearby.

DISCUSSING THE PROCEDURE WITH THE PATIENT

Before performing the biopsy, it is very important to spend a sufficient amount of time discussing the procedure with the patient. Breathing instructions should be explained well in advance and before the administration of any conscious sedation. The importance of the patient's cooperation must be strongly emphasized, and the procedure must be explained in a way that the average nonmedical citizen can understand. The risks and potential complications must be explained along with a realistic assessment of the likelihood of untoward events such as pneumothorax, hemoptysis, air embolism, and any other special risks that apply to specific patients. Postprocedural and periprocedural preventative measures such as puncture site down-positioning and the placement of a blood patch should also be explained. If a patient is at increased risk of developing a complication, a thorough preprocedure explanation of the possible untoward events will help the patient remain calm if a complication does occur.

Patient comfort is extremely important to allow the appropriate biopsy position to be maintained. Supine patients are more comfortable with their arms at their sides, whereas prone patients are most comfortable with their arms placed under their head and the head turned to one side. Decubitus positions are used only if absolutely necessary because the lateral decubitus positions predispose to greater patient movement. Various positioning equipment such as straps, blankets, wedges, pillows, and arm rests should be employed to help keep the patient comfortable and motionless throughout the procedure.

Given that percutaneous lung biopsy requires active participation by the patient if the procedure is to be reliably successful, it is optimally done under local anesthesia alone. The patient will be better able to follow breathing instructions and better able to report any postprocedural symptoms that may occur. Despite this rationale, the amount of perceived pain and discomfort varies widely between patients, and conscious sedation may be necessary for the patient to tolerate the procedure. One method of approaching the procedure is to begin with only local anesthetic and give additional sedation and/or pain medication as is necessary.

Risk Factors and Complications

The primary complications in lung biopsy are pneumothorax, hemoptysis, and air embolism. The risk of a pneumothorax is increased by the presence of obstructive lung disease, and a direct puncture of a superficial bulla will usually result in the rapid development of a pneumothorax. The risk of pulmonary hemorrhage is increased by abnormal clotting factors, inadequate or dysfunctional platelets (thrombocytopenia, renal failure, aspirin), pulmonary hypertension, and the biopsy of inherently vascular lesions (i.e., carcinoid tumors, vascular metastases, chronic inflammatory cavities). Lung biopsy is not advisable when there is abnormal clotting function approaching therapeutic anticoagulation (i.e., INR > 1.3) or when the platelet count is less than 100,000/mL. When biopsy is necessary, despite an increase risk of hemorrhage, a single pass into a lesion using a small-gage needle is recommended, and avoiding the use of core biopsy needles in these patients is advisable. The risk of air embolism is increased in an uncooperative patient primarily owing to a deep or rapid inspiration when the inner cannula of the needle is open to air and the needle tip happens to be within a pulmonary vein. Air embolism is also increased with positive pressure ventilation. Average complication rates for lung biopsy range from 10 to 20% for pneumothoraces, 4 to 5% for hemoptysis, and <1% for air embolism.

Most other contraindications to lung biopsy are relative and must be weighed against the potential benefits that may be gained from performing the biopsy. An option in high-risk patients (other than refusing to perform the biopsy), is to plan the procedure to maximize patient safety. This includes preprocedure preparation in anticipation of the complications most likely to occur.

The Biopsy Target

Various criteria are used to select the most appropriate biopsy target and to predict the success of the procedure. When multiple lesions are present, both size and location are important in choosing exactly which lesion is the most appropriate in terms of patient safety and likelihood of obtaining diagnostic material. For example, a smaller lesion may be preferable to a larger lesion if the location is more favorable. Overall, most lesions 1 cm or larger are amenable to percutaneous biopsy in all except the most unfavorable of locations.

The ideal target is a lung lesion that lies adjacent to the chest wall with a nonaerated pathway to biopsy the lesion (Fig. 8A). If the biopsy can be accomplished through nonaerated lung, the risk of a pneumothorax is significantly decreased.

The position of the lesion within the lung is important, as lower lung nodules move significantly more with respiration than upper lung nodules. In the absence of real-time imaging, a relatively small lower lung lesion can be much more challenging to sample than a lesion of similar size in the upper lung. The lower the lesion is within the lung, the more important the patient's breathing cooperation becomes if the procedure is to be successful.

Pleural-based lesions adjacent to the chest wall are usually preferable to sample because of the decreased risk of pneumothorax. If no pleural-based lesions are available, a larger relatively peripheral lesion is the preferred target. The puncture site and trajectory should be directed toward the center of the lesion, and the needle should be oriented as straight vertically or horizontally as possible. The direct vertical or horizontal orientation of the needle will aid in visually keeping the needle correctly oriented while performing the biopsy. Biopsy of small, deep lesions is associated with more complications because of longer procedure times and more needle manipulation and should be avoided unless another lesion more amenable to biopsy is not present.

The ideal location for a small nodule target is toward the periphery of the lung but not immediately subjacent to the visceral pleura. This will allow the physician to avoid the larger deep pulmonary vessels and the pleural space while providing enough anatomic space for redirection of the needle after the initial pleural puncture. Small lesions that are in difficult locations can be very challenging to sample successfully. Small subpleural lesions, for example, are difficult to biopsy without causing a pneumothorax. Small lesions adjacent to the heart or great vessels are generally not appropriate for biopsy unless a tangential approach is possible or CT fluoroscopy is available. Lesions just inferior to the minor fissure may also be difficult to sample without violating the interlobar fissure itself, and lesions deep in the costophrenic angle region of the lungs may move significantly with respiration, predisposing to injuries of

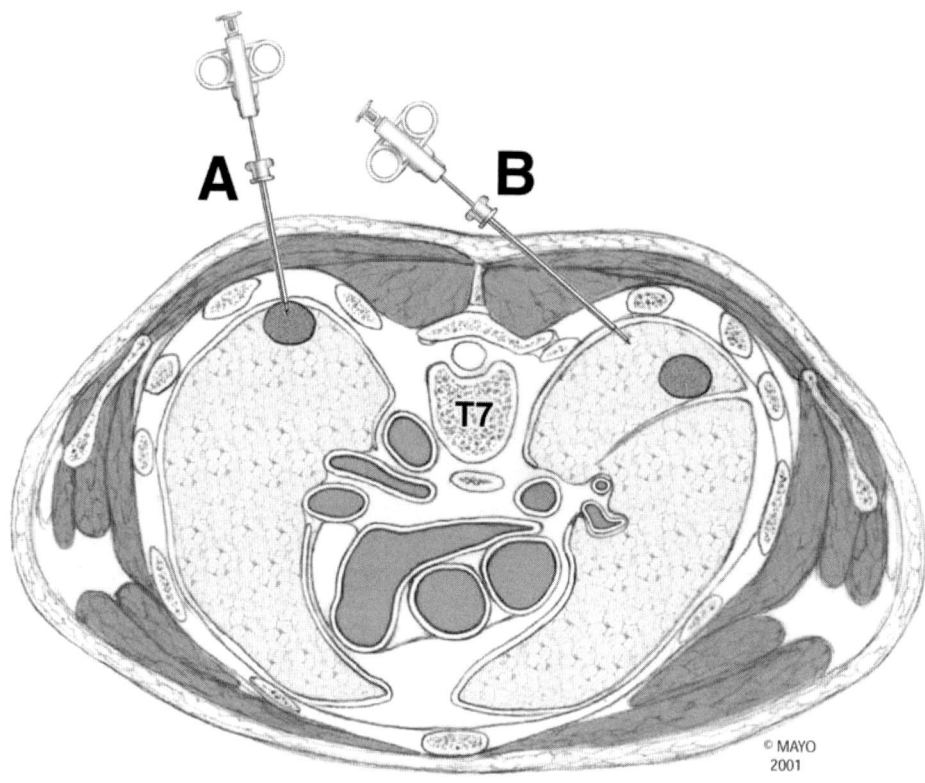

Fig. 8. Biopsy of peripheral pulmonary lesions.

(A) If a pulmonary nodule is accessible through nonaerated lung, that is the preferable pathway. If the guiding needle cannot be secured within the nodule, the outer cannula can recoil into the pleural space, producing a pneumothorax. If a subpleural nodule cannot be biopsied using a direct approach, a tangential approach may be required.

(B) The tangential approach traverses more aerated lung but decreases the risk of pneumothorax caused by the outer cannula recoiling into the pleural space.

the associated hemidiaphragm or underlying structures. Very small lesions (smaller than 5–6 mm) in general are unlikely to yield diagnostic material and should be approached with caution.

When no critical structures obstruct the pathway to the pulmonary lesion and when no interlobar fissures will be crossed, a posterior biopsy approach is the most optimal choice for many reasons. This technique has been associated with a decreased pneumothorax rate, and the postprocedure biopsy side-down position is easier for the patient when he or she is lying on the back rather than in a prone position. The prone patient also does not have the opportunity to view the long needles, blood, and other parts of the biopsy procedure that might be distressing. If the patient cannot maintain the prone position either during the biopsy or afterwards, a lateral approach is the trajectory of choice.

A prior thoracotomy will also reduce the risk of pneumothorax because of the adherent pleural surfaces that result from postoperative scarring. If a patient has multiple bilateral lesions of approximately the same size, and the exact site of the prior surgery can be adequately avoided, then the side of the previous thoracotomy is the preferred side for lung biopsy.

Biopsy of mediastinal or hilar lesions must be approached cautiously, and a high-quality CT examination with iv contrast can assist in defining vasculature or other structures that should be avoided. It is important to avoid the systemic and pulmonary arteries owing to the risk of hemorrhage, and it is also important to avoid the pulmonary veins because of the possibility of air embolism. Despite adequate preprocedural planning and an optimal equipment armamentarium, some parts of the mediastinal area may be inaccessible. For example, small nodes in the precarinal area interposed between the trachea and the transverse portion of the aortic arch are generally not amenable to a percutaneous approach.

Plotting the Course

Extrapulmonary Route

If the aerated portion of the lung is not entered, there will be no risk of pneumothorax, and lesions that are pleural based should be biopsied while attempting to avoid the air-filled portions of the lung. Other opportunities to avoid entering the lung include crossing atelectatic or consolidated lung. If a central mass causing peripheral obstruction is difficult to separate from

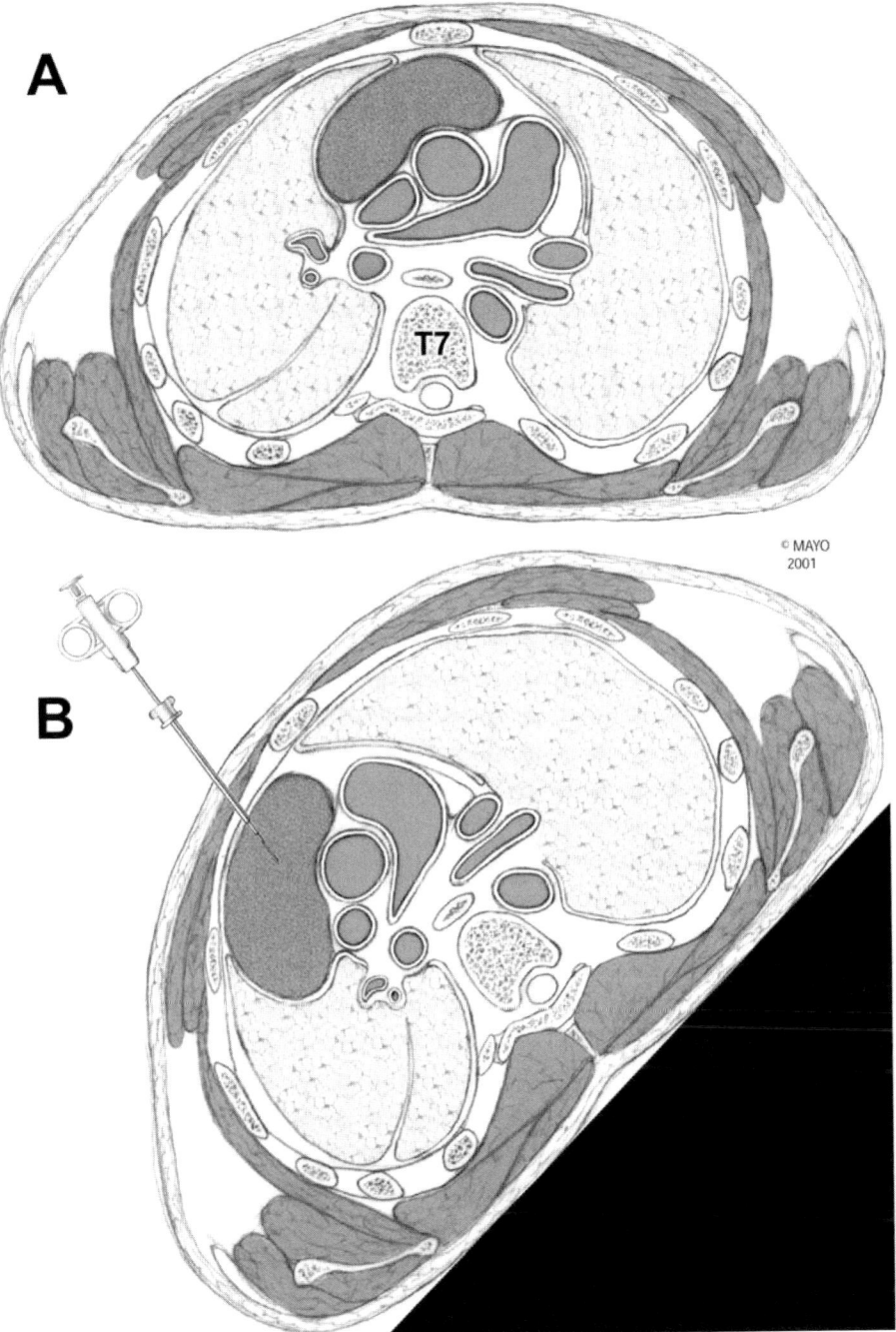

Fig. 9. Mediastinal biopsy. When a biopsy of a mediastinal mass is performed, it is desirable to avoid traversing the pleura or osseous structures. The mediastinum moves with alterations in patient position, and this phenomenon can be used to one's advantage during mediastinal biopsy. The illustrated patient's anterior mediastinal mass (**A**) becomes more accessible when the patient is placed in a steep, right posterior oblique position; (**B**) thereby allowing porcutaneous access to the mass without the risk of traversing the pleura, lung, or sternum.

the atelectatic lung, a contrast-enhanced CT scan of the region will improve identification of the mass and will help avoid sampling errors caused by biopsying atelectatic lung or obstructive pneumonia.

If possible, accessing mediastinal lesions without entering the lung is the most optimal approach. The mediastinum is mobile, and positioning the patient in an oblique or decubitus position may move structures from behind the bony thorax and create a pathway to the mediastinal lesion *(Fig. 9)*. Access to mediastinal or lung lesions may also be achieved with a paraspinal approach. If necessary, saline or a saline/lidocaine mixture may be injected into the paravertebral soft tissues to widen the extrapleural soft tissue pathway. Injection into the extrapleural space must be approached with caution, as this could produce vagal stimulation. Although the SVC and innominate veins may be transgressed with a thin needle, this route is not advisable in some patients. Access to the middle mediastinum may also be obtained through the thoracic inlet, but this technique is difficult and requires additional training to master.

Each patient should be considered individually when deciding on the particular route of access to the mediastinum, whether the pathway transgresses the lungs or other structures. Most of the more invasive techniques such as saline/lidocaine instillation or thoracic inlet access should not be used in patients with severe illnesses, in the elderly, or in those with problematic cardiac disease: these techniques have a propensity to cause vasovagal stimulation. The hypotension and bradycardia that often accompany this stimulation can have adverse and serious effects on those patients less able to tolerate the decreased cardiac output.

Pulmonary Route

With most lung lesions, a variety of pathways may be considered. It is preferable to make the pleural puncture with the needle oriented perpendicular to the visceral pleura, as there is less of a chance that the needle tip will slide over the outer pleural surface, resulting in an unexpected intrapulmonary needle position. Interlobar fissures should also be avoided since such transgression results in three punctures of the pleural surfaces rather than one. This will increase the risk of a pneumothorax over a single visceral pleural puncture.

For small, subpleural lesions, a direct puncture may not be appropriate owing to the increased risk of pneumothorax and the limited distance available to redirect the needle after its insertion into the lung. To avoid these hazards, a tangential approach *(Fig. 8B)* provides access to the lesion, affords the necessary space for needle adjustment, and makes it less likely that the needle tip will be withdrawn to rest in the pleural space.

When passing though the chest wall, a course should be plotted that passes over the adjacent rib rather than under it. The neurovascular bundle courses around the rib at its inferior margin and may be injured when a needle is placed through this location. This approach is less important in the anterior chest wall since both the arteries and veins decrease in caliber as they pass anteriorly. The needle should also avoid direct contact with the rib itself since the periosteal irritation may cause pain resulting in vagal stimulation, and the needle will be more difficult to redirect if placed directly adjacent to a rib. The ribs appear as elliptical or oval on axial CT images. The ribs are oriented inferiorly as they course anteriorly, and therefore the superior edge of the rib is the end of the oval farthest away from the spine. The inferior edge of the rib (the location that should be avoided) is the portion of the oval nearest to the spine.

During the initial evaluation to determine the most appropriate biopsy pathway, a rib may be found that blocks the desired trajectory of the needle path. Various techniques may be used to solve this problem, including moving the puncture site more medially or laterally, adjusting the needle angle, puncturing from the opposite side of the patient, rotating the patient into a slightly decubitus position, or angling the CT gantry (to allow image guidance with superior or inferior angulation of the needle). Although a transosseous approach is possible, this should be a technique of last resort, and needles designed for the transosseous portion of the procedure should be used to augment the traditional lung biopsy armamentarium.

Evaluation of the Biopsy Site

Although conventional fluoroscopy has been a time-tested method of lung biopsy, CT has the advantage of providing detailed cross-sectional anatomy when evaluating the exact site that is to be biopsied. Thin-section CT can be valuable in locating the exact site of puncture that can be appropriately placed in the interspaces between the ribs. Thin sections are also useful in evaluating the condition of the lung parenchyma and for the presence of emphysema, bullae, or blebs. Given that only the puncture site leaks air and that air does not track along the pulmonary interstitium after biopsy, entering the lung where the parenchyma is the most normal is important. Traversing bullae or other abnormal structures deeper within the lung is not considered a risk factor for developing a pneumothorax. The lung should be entered in a region that is more normal in appearance and, even in patients with severe lung disease, there is usually a region of more normal-appearing lung that would be an appropriate pulmonary puncture site.

Traversing a bleb or bulla, especially one that is large, usually results in a pneumothorax and sometimes causes a persistent air leak. If severely diseased lung must be traversed, some experts would advocate that a small-gage chest tube be placed prophylactically, and others would advocate that a chest tube be placed in an optimal location just outside the parietal pleura. Regardless of the approach, a high-flow air leak caused by the puncture of a bleb can result in patient extremis and can necessitate the emergent placement of a chest tube. Adequate preparation for thoracostomy tube placement in these patients may allow a more rapid and efficient tube placement.

The phase of respiration is also important when evaluating the pulmonary target. Ideally, a small to medium inspiration is the desired lung volume for a lung biopsy breath hold. A lung puncture in deep inspiration or end expiration puts stress on the pleura at the puncture site, especially when the needle is left in place (coaxial technique). This can result in a pleural tear and a persistent air leak. The level of comfort is also much higher when the patient is allowed to take a comfortable breath in, rather than to hold the respiration repeatedly at the extreme ranges of breathing. When biopsies, by necessity, are done in expiration, great care must be taken to avoid patient inspiration during the sampling process. When the patient is holding the breath in expiration, the natural tendency is to take in a breath at the earliest possible time. This significantly increases the risk of developing an air embolus, which places the patient at higher risk.

The Biopsy

After the procedure has been explained, the biopsy target selected, the trajectory planned, and the patient instructed how to breathe, the local anesthetic is given using sterile technique. Lidocaine (1–1.5%) is infiltrated into the skin and subcutaneous soft tissues while the patient is instructed to hold the designated level of inspiration. The anesthetic should be delivered up to the pleura, but care should be taken not to puncture the parietal pleura during the delivery of anesthesia. After the delivery of anesthesia, the appropriate needle position is confirmed by using the lidocaine needle as a guide. A very small skin incision made at the biopsy site by a pointed scalpel or other sharp blade will facilitate needle entry. Excessive bleeding after the small skin incision should call additional attention to the patient's clotting status and may necessitate termination of the procedure if a problem with coagulation is found.

When using a coaxial system, the length that the inner needle will extend distally from the outer cannula (the pass length) should be set before the procedure. The stylet is removed from the outer cannula, and the inner needle is inserted through the lumen of the outer cannula (*Fig. 7A*). The desired length that the inner needle will protrude from the distal tip of the outer cannula is then set with a plastic marker (usually found on the inner needle and used for this purpose). Most core biopsy needles will also have such a marker, and the pass length can be set exactly the same way. Many core biopsy needles have adjustable throw lengths as well, and this should also be adjusted before beginning the biopsy procedure. Later, during the procedure, the pass length and the throw length can be adjusted if necessary.

The outer needle of the coaxial system is inserted into the soft tissues of the chest wall far enough to allow the needle to maintain its position without holding it. In thin patients or patients with suboptimal thoracic muscular tone, a limited amount of extrapleural soft tissue may be available. Whenever the angle of the needle is not maintained by surrounding soft tissues, the needle can be stabilized by a long clamp (if CT fluoroscopy is used) or by a combination of gauze pads, tape, and sterile towels. Plastic needle holders are also available that will stabilize the needle in a predetermined position outside the skin.

Care should be taken when advancing the needle to remain in the scan plane of the CT gantry. The outer cannula should be placed just outside the parietal pleura. Positioning the needle tip in this location is very important, as the patient's musculature can cause substantial redirection of the needle when advancement is attempted from the skin to an intrapulmonary location. When the needle is positioned just outside the parietal pleura, it can be directed at the lesion, and the patient can be tested for the ability to reproduce the designated respiration. If the patient is not breathing as instructed previously, additional instructions may be given as the patient's breathing is observed. All needle

manipulations, even within the chest wall, should be performed with the patient holding the breath in the manner discussed with him or her before the procedure. The simple motion of respiration can move the chest wall significantly, and the appropriate angulation of the needle cannot be maintained if the appropriate level of inspiration cannot be reproduced consistently.

The entry of the needle through the pleura causes sharp pain, and the patient should be warned that this will happen so they can anticipate the pain and not react with a sudden movement. After entry into the lung, the needle should not be manipulated unless the patient is holding the breath at the predetermined level of inspiration. After the needle is inserted into the lung, it should be allowed to move freely with respiration. Any maneuvering of the needle while the patient is breathing increases the risk of a pleural tear and subsequent pneumothorax.

When the needle is manipulated, the nondominant hand should hold the distal needle (nearest the skin), and the dominant hand should hold the proximal end of the needle. This technique will allow the needle to be passed though tissue that is fibrous or noncompliant and facilitates redirection of the needle by using the proximal hand as a pivot point.

When the needle is inserted into the lung, it should be advanced at least 1–2 cm into the lung parenchyma regardless of the depth of the lung lesion. Because of the significant movement of the lungs during normal breathing (especially in the lower lungs), this amount of transgression is necessary to keep the needle from moving proximally into the pleural space. With ideal positioning, the needle will be passed through the lesion and can be retracted to a point near the proximal portion of the lesion. The coaxial pass length can then be adjusted to equal the size of the lesion distal to the tip of the outer cannula, and multiple biopsies can be taken.

Deep lung lesions can be accessed by incremental advancement of the needle, monitoring of the needle position, and *ad hoc* adjustment of the needle position based on the size and location of the target. Monitoring of the needle tip location should be done with 5-mm sections (1–2 mm sections are useful for small lung lesions). When the coaxial technique is used, very small lesions may be pushed away by the outer cannula. A smaller needle, however, placed through the outer cannula can usually be placed into the nodule and used to sample these small lesions.

Obtaining Tissue

After access to the pulmonary lesion is obtained, the pass length and the throw length of the needles should be reexamined to ensure that any sampling of normal lung is minimized. In addition to not being diagnostically helpful, sampling normal lung increases the risk of hemorrhage. Adequately planned pass lengths will also help the physician to avoid other obstacles such as fissures, vessels, and mediastinal structures.

Obtaining tissue requires both hands. The nondominant hand is used to stabilize the outer needle (which is held only after the patient has suspended respiration). The inner stylet is removed, and sampling is performed with the dominant hand. Constant suction is helpful during the sampling process, and pulling back the plunger with one's thumb can generate strong suction force. Suction of air into the syringe indicates that normal lung is being sampled or that there is a poor connection between the syringe and the needle. Short forceful thrusts are used to obtain tissue, and five rapid thrusts are usually made unless a significant amount of blood appears within the syringe. If this occurs, additional passes will further dilute the specimen, and no additional passes should be performed in obtaining that particular specimen. After the sampling process, the stylet is replaced, and the patient is instructed to resume normal respiration.

The size and appearance of the specimen that is retrieved may provide valuable information. The lesion may feel firm or scirrhous, characteristics typical of malignancies, or the lesion may feel very firm or rubbery. If the lesion is firm and the operator has the sensation that the lesion is being pushed away rather than being punctured, a thinner needle or a core biopsy needle may be necessary for successful sampling. If the biopsy needle is appropriately positioned in relation to the target and does not yield any pathologic tissue after a few passes, then the lesion could be benign. Also, if no tissue is obtained despite adequate positioning, the lesion is also more likely benign given that neoplastic processes tend to be loosely adherent and are most often easily aspirated. Strong consideration should be given to obtaining core biopsy samples, as some lesions such as fibrous tumors of the pleura and many benign lesions are unlikely to be diagnosed with aspiration biopsy. If core biopsy is planned, the outer needle for a coaxial core biopsy setup can be used to obtain both the aspiration and core biopsy samples. This technique will avoid a second pleural puncture and is suitable for obtaining both types of biopsies.

During the process of obtaining tissue, the outer needle may change position. Therefore, the tip of the outer cannula should be reimaged after each coaxial pass. If an on-site pathologist is present and routinely renders a preliminary analysis, this time can be used to determine the position of the tip of the outer cannula and confirm its position. The images obtained will also provide information about whether the patient has developed a pneumothorax or parenchymal hemorrhage.

The coaxial technique is especially useful in allowing multiple biopsies to be obtained quickly and without an additional pleural puncture. This technique is especially useful when a larger amount of tissue is needed or when cytologic services are not available at the time of the biopsy. Many passes can be made, lessening the chance that the procedure will not yield adequate material. Also, if a favorable pathway to the pulmonary lesion is present, it is unusual to have a pneumothorax with the coaxial technique even during long procedures. This is primarily owing to the limited number of pleural punctures (usually one) and the fact that the needle itself occludes the puncture site during the procedure. Even if a pneumothorax develops, the needle tip will usually remain lodged within the lesion, allowing more biopsies to be obtained.

When performing biopsies of a pulmonary lesion, the hub of the needle may be moved in a small circular pattern, thus directing the needle tip in a slightly different location. This will allow biopsies to be taken in somewhat different locations within the lesion. When multiple different biopsies are needed from different areas within the same lesion, a side exit coaxial system is also available that can sample different areas just by turning the needle before obtaining the biopsy.

The biopsy procedure is concluded when an adequate pathologic specimen is obtained, a symptomatic pneumothorax develops, there is severe hemorrhage/hemoptysis, or the patient requests that the procedure be terminated.

Correction of Unsatisfactory Needle Position

Despite meticulous planning and appropriate technique, the initial needle placement may be either suboptimal or may miss the pulmonary lesion entirely. Given the increased risk of pneumothorax with multiple pleural punctures, corrective manipulations of the needle should be performed by withdrawing the needle and redirecting it without making a second puncture though the visceral pleura. The outer cannula of a coaxial system is usually fairly stiff and is amenable to redirection in the vast majority of patients. Often, the necessary amount of corrective angulation that is needed appears to be an overexaggeration, and the operator should not be surprised if significant needle angulation is required to alter the original needle orientation. The redirection of the needle can be facilitated by placing the dominant hand on the proximal end of the needle, using the nondominant hand at the skin's surface as a fulcrum, and using the bevel of the needle to direct the tip toward the lesion (Fig. 10A).

Needle redirection in obese patients may be especially difficult because the large amount of soft tissue in the thorax tends to preserve the needle's original trajectory. Whenever the needle is inserted to the hub, it is also more difficult to redirect and a longer needle should be used in obese patients when it is possible to fit the longer needle length into the CT gantry. If the needle is placed superior or inferior to the target, it may be withdrawn to the lung periphery and redirected after the patient has performed expiration or inspiration maneuvers. The changes in respiration level may bring the lesion in line with the needle and allow the needle to be advanced directly into the target.

If a single-beveled needle is used, the needle can be directed using the bevel angle to direct the needle. In soft tissue and in the lung (to a lesser degree), the needle tends to angle slightly toward the direction of the pointed tip and away from the face of the bevel (Fig. 10B). Appropriate bevel positioning can augment the other maneuvers listed above to facilitate redirection of the needle. Additionally, if a difficult needle angle is anticipated before the procedure a slight bend may be placed in the needle coincident with the bevel of the needle 0.5–1.0 cm from the tip (Fig. 10C). This allows much greater steerability of the needle, especially though the soft tissues, but this technique should be used only if the operator is comfortable with the increased needle deflection that this bend will provide. The needle point can also be used to pierce the pleura when approaching a lesion tangentially. With the bevel face directed

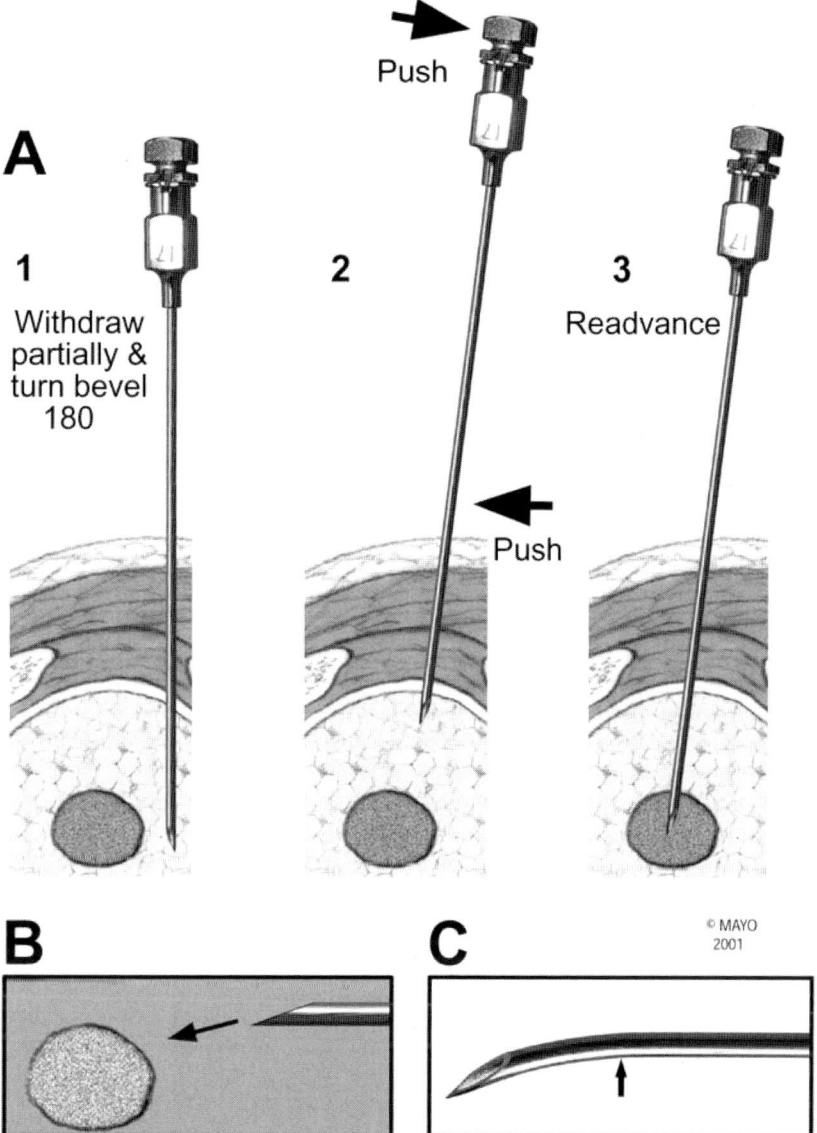

Fig. 10. Correction of an unsatisfactory needle position.

(A) 1. The needle is withdrawn proximal to the lesion but not proximal to the visceral pleura. The face of the bevel is rotated away from the lesion to facilitate needle movement toward the target.

2. The hub of the needle is pushed in the direction needed to correct the trajectory of the needle. Additional leverage may be applied by pushing the distal portion of the needle (just superficial to the skin) in the opposite direction.

3. The needle is readvanced into the lesion.

(B) The bevel of the needle should face away from the desired direction of the needle. By using this method, the needle's natural tendency to move slightly away from the face of the bevel can be used to one's advantage in directing the needle toward a specific target.

(C) A slight bend in the needle placed 0.5–1.0 cm from the tip of and coincident with the bevel causes the needle to deflect more away from the face of the bevel. This provides a much greater ability to steer the needle by directing the notch of the needle's hub (usually placed on the same side of the needle as the face of the bevel) away from the desired direction of the needle.

away from the outer surface of the lung, the needle point will be directed toward the center of the lung and will tend to penetrate the pleural surfaces, thereby allowing the needle to pass into the lung parenchyma. Before beginning the biopsy, the operator should examine the needle and note the position of the locking hub and notch at the proximal end of the needle and the relationship of the proximal notch to the needle's bevel angle distally. Most often the notch will be on the same side as the face of the bevel. The natural tendency of the needle, therefore, will be to steer away from the notch. The operator should remain cognizant of the anatomy of the needle and use it to advantage throughout the procedure.

In some cases, despite multiple different techniques and attempts at needle repositioning, adequate repositioning of the outer needle is not possible. The operator can pull the outer needle back to the periphery of the pulmonary lesion and correct the faulty angulation during the tissue sampling process with the patient holding the breath. Although this is not an optimal approach to sampling lung lesions, it is often effective, and a second pleural puncture can be avoided.

When the original needle position is too far away from the desired location that is cannot be corrected, a second pleural puncture is necessary. While attempting the second puncture, the first needle should be left in place and should remain there until the procedure has been completed. The presence of the first needle will block air leakage from the original first puncture site and will fix the local position of the lung, making additional punctures less susceptible to respiratory motion.

Cytology

Immediate cytologic feedback from an on-site pathologist is an ideal situation when a transthoracic biopsy is performed. Rapid staining techniques (i.e., toluidine blue stain) and an experienced pathologist can provide accurate results in 2–3 min after the biopsy specimen is obtained. Confirmation of adequate sampling can shorten procedure time, allow for radiologist/pathologist exchange of information, and increase the yield of the procedure. If the tissue obtained is not sufficiently cellular, additional material can be obtained or the needle may be directed to a different portion of the lesion. If tissue necrosis is seen, the needle can be directed toward the periphery of the lesion. Abundant inflammatory cells indicate that specimens should be taken for culture, and some fungi can also be identified using rapid staining techniques.

Gross visual inspection is an inaccurate assessment of the adequacy of the biopsy. Relatively large amounts of tissue may be obtained that give little diagnostic information, whereas a single pass through representative tissue can produce an accurate diagnosis. If a pathologist or cytotechnologist is not available, the physician performing the biopsy may want to become familiar with the essential components of cytologic examination including smear technique, fixation of the specimen, and identification of the features typical of neoplasia. Familiarity with some of the nonneoplastic findings such as organizing pneumonia, granulomatous changes, and normal bronchial cells is also helpful when analyzing the biopsy specimen to determine the adequacy of the tissue required.

Safety Precautions

Pneumothorax Prevention

If aerated lung has not been transgressed, the risk of the patient developing a pneumothorax is negligible. Otherwise, even with appropriate technique and meticulous adherence to the various safety measures, the risk of the patient developing a pneumothorax remains. An additional measure designed to prevent the development of a pneumothorax is known as the blood patch technique. This technique can only be used with a coaxial biopsy approach and involves using the patient's own blood to prevent air leakage from the pleural puncture. The original blood patch technique described the use of clotted blood injected through the biopsy track, but most individuals use blood drawn directly from the patient's arm (usually from the saline lock). Approx 5–7 mL of blood is taken from the patient and injected through the outer cannula of the coaxial biopsy apparatus. The outer needle is pulled back to within 1.5–3.0 cm of the visceral pleura, and the blood is injected as the needle is slowly withdrawn through the pleura and into the chest wall.

Objective evidence that the blood patch technique provides additional protection against developing a pneumothorax originates from lung biopsy models showing that most patched lungs require higher intrapulmonary pressures before air leakage is observed. On average, the pressure required to cause leakage in patched lungs is twice that of lungs that are not patched. Despite this effectiveness, the blood patch technique will not be helpful when the air leak is caused by a large pleural laceration.

The blood patch should be delivered in the peripheral 1.5–3.0 cm of the lung since this will prevent a leak in the visceral pleura, where pneumothoraces develop. Injection of blood into the deep parenchyma of the lung will have little to no effect in preventing a pneumothorax. Also, injections of fresh blood deep in the lung increases the chance that a small blood clot could enter a pulmonary vein and embolize into the systemic arterial system. Injection of blood in the portion of the lung containing only tiny vessels makes the chance of embolism negligible.

Placing the patient in a biopsy-site-down position after biopsy will facilitate the blood placement at or near the pleural puncture site. The freshly drawn blood should then clot at this site, forming a seal within the prior biopsy track.

Other pleural patching options have been utilized including a method that involves injecting gelatin sponge particles into the biopsy track. Both the blood patch and gelatin sponge options have met with varying degrees of success. The existing literature also reports mixed results for pleural patching techniques, but larger, more definitive studies still have not been completed comparing the various techniques with each other and with patients without pleural patching procedures.

When Complications Occur

Pneumothorax

Small pneumothoraces are relatively common, and many patients will experience sharp, pleuritic-type chest pain. During the procedure the patient's blood oxygen saturation should be measured. This will allow detection of hypoxemia if a significant pneumothorax develops. The size of a pneumothorax that will cause shortness of breath varies significantly between patients and is dependent on factors such as preexisting lung disease, comorbidity, and overall physical condition.

If a small pneumothorax develops during the procedure, an additional hour in the puncture-side-down position is recommended. The patient's oxygen saturation and vital signs should be monitored, high-flow oxygen (by facemask) should be delivered, and a chest X-ray should be obtained after the extra hour of puncture-side-down positioning. If the pneumothorax has not increased in size, the patient is allowed to sit up for the next hour without the oxygen. If the pneumothorax remains unchanged or decreased in size, the patient may be discharged. If the pneumothorax has increased in size, the patient is returned to the puncture-side-down position for another hour, and the process is repeated. This sequence of events continues until the patient is either prepared for discharge or requires placement of a thoracostomy tube. Signs that the patient requires tube placement include a large pneumothorax (i.e., greater than 30%), persistent pleural air leak, or the appearance of symptoms from the pneumothorax.

Pneumothoraces may appear atypical in patients with prior infection, surgery, or radiation therapy. In general, patients with prior injury or inflammation of the pleural space are less likely to develop pneumothoraces. When they occur, however, the appearance can be atypical and must be recognized as a pneumothorax if the patient is to receive the appropriate therapy and/or supportive measures.

Aspiration of a Pneumothorax

Patients developing a pneumothorax during a lung biopsy procedure may undergo percutaneous aspiration of the air within the pleural space. This technique will not help those patients with a moderate to large size pleural tear but may avert the need for chest tube patients in a large portion of patients.

A needle with a sharp center stylet and a relatively blunt outer cannula can be used for pneumothorax aspiration. These needles are effective at aspirating the excess air but do not kink like many pleural catheters and are less likely to damage the visceral pleura when the collapsed lung is reexpanded. A 17–20-g needle can be used for aspiration and connected directly to wall suction via a pressure limited suction apparatus. A 50–60 mL syringe with a three-way stopcock may also be used for aspiration but requires more manipulation and is slower than automated suction.

The needle tip is placed just internal to the parietal pleura, and the inner stylet is removed. The needle hub is promptly placed to suction, and the air within the pleural space is evacuated. If a pneumothorax occurs during a biopsy, the outer cannula of the coaxial biopsy apparatus may be used, and the aspiration can occur after the blood patch has been placed in the outer portion of the collapsed lung.

If needle aspiration is not completely effective at reexpanding the lung, it may also be used as a provisional solution until a larger thoracostomy tube is placed. This technique is usually effective at alleviating a symptomatic patient's shortness of breath until a pleural drainage tube can be placed under less emergent circumstances.

When a pleural drainage tube is required, a small-diameter tube (i.e., 9–10 Fr) is usually quite sufficient in reexpanding the lung. Larger tubes are not necessary unless more extensive pleural drainage is required. The chest tube may be placed either in the midaxillary line or in the midclavicular line, and levels from the 2nd to the 6th intercostal spaces have been described. The operator must take care not to injure underlying structures such as the diaphragm and heart and must avoid making direct contact with the apical pleural surfaces, as tube tip placement in this location can be painful for the patient. If pleural fluid is encountered, the operator should consider placing a larger diameter tube, as the smaller 9–10-Fr tubes can become obstructed with pleural space debris or clotted blood. Patients requiring thoracostomy tubes need hospital admission and observation. Continuous suction is the preferred method of lung expansion, and this should be applied overnight. The following morning, the tube is left in place and clamped for 1 h. An expiratory chest film is obtained after the tube has been clamped for an hour, and, if no pneumothorax is present, the tube is removed. An immediate post chest tube removal film is obtained, and the patient is monitored for an additional hour. At this time additional inspiration and expiration chest films are obtained and if no pneumothorax is present, the patient may be discharged. If a pneumothorax is present and is larger compared with the postremoval film, the patient is again placed in the puncture-side-down position and given oxygen by facemask; then postbiopsy therapy for a small pneumothorax is reinitiated. If the pneumothorax is large or the lung has collapsed completely, the chest tube is reinserted and the process repeated.

HEMOPTYSIS

Hemoptysis occurs in approx 5–10% of lung biopsies and is usually self-limiting. Although hemoptysis is most often a minor complication; it can be severe in certain patients and remains one of the leading causes of death in lung biopsies. Massive hemoptysis can result from the laceration of enlarged bronchial arteries that may be present in patients with such conditions as chronic obstructive lung disease, inflammatory cavities, and bronchiectasis. Most hemoptysis, however, results from trauma to the pulmonary arteries or veins surrounding the biopsy target.

Early indicators that will alert the operator to the presence of pulmonary hemorrhage include bleeding though the outer needle of the coaxial biopsy set or increasing density surrounding the biopsy target as seen at fluoroscopy or on CT. If these findings are present, prudent actions include limiting the amount of needle manipulation, keeping the biopsy time to a minimum, and maintaining a heightened awareness of the patient's vital signs. Unfortunately, pulmonary hemorrhage is also a significant irritant to the airways and can induce spasmodic coughing in the patient undergoing the biopsy. Vigorous coughing with the biopsy needle in place can cause a pleural tear or an air embolism if the deep inspiration before the cough happens to draw air into the pulmonary venous system through the needle. Persistent severe coughing, therefore, is an indication for biopsy needle removal.

If the pulmonary hemorrhage is persistent or brisk, the patient should be placed in the decubitus position with the biopsy side down to prevent the hemorrhage from spreading to the contralateral lung. The patient should be allowed to expectorate the hemorrhage and will do this reflexively, as the blood will stimulate the cough reflex. If possible, intubation should be avoided but, if necessary, should be performed with a double-lumen tube. An individual experienced in the placement of this type of tube should perform the intubation procedure if possible. If the hemorrhage does not stop with expectant management, bronchoscopic tamponade of the lobar bronchus is the treatment of choice. Other options include bronchial artery embolization (if this is the source of bleeding), segmental pulmonary artery embolization, and thoracotomy. Appropriate surgical support is very important and should be available if a complication develops that cannot be treated percutaneously.

AIR EMBOLISM

Entry of air into the pulmonary venous system with subsequent systemic air embolization can result in very serious complications related to cerebral infarction. As mentioned previously, air embolization may occur if the patient inspires when the needle tip is located within a pulmonary vein and the inner stylet has been removed. The creation of a bronchovenous fistula may also occur during the biopsy procedure owing to local trauma to these structures. This may occur at any location along the biopsy track where the needle has damaged both structures lying in close proximity to each other.

When the embolization occurs, patients may exhibit signs of seizure activity or stroke. They may also become significantly disoriented or lose consciousness. An immediate response is required: delivery of 100% oxygen (by facemask) and placing the patient in a Trendelenburg position. These actions will facilitate absorption of the nitrogen-containing bubbles within the cerebral arterial circulation, and the Trendelenburg positioning should prevent any further air from exiting the left atrium and reaching the systemic circulation. If Trendelenburg positioning cannot be performed, placing the patient in a left lateral decubitus position will decrease the risk of systemic air embolization. If bronchovenous fistula is suspected as a cause of the air embolization, intubation and mechanical ventilation should be avoided, as positive pressure ventilation will exacerbate the problem.

After the Procedure

Monitoring

Postbiopsy care directly influences the development and severity of complications associated with transthoracic lung biopsy. While traditionally not thought of as postprocedure care, certain immediate postbiopsy activities are vitally important in terms of patient management and to prevent complications. For example, most pneumothoraces occur at or around the time of needle removal, and most cases of hemoptysis begin near the end of the procedure.

Immediately after the procedure, the patient should be placed in a biopsy-side-down position and transferred to the gurney when it is conveniently available. The staff should do the transfer as the patient remains passive, to avoid increasing intrathoracic pressure. If some assistance by the patient is required, he or she may roll onto the gurney while exhaling to prevent an inadvertent Valsalva maneuver and the resultant increased pleural stress. The monitoring process should continue throughout this transfer, and close attention is warranted to search for the early signs of complications. Vital signs should be obtained every 15 min for the first hour, and the patient's oxygen saturation should be monitored. Vital signs should be taken more frequently if the patient becomes unstable and if a pneumothorax is present; oxygen may be provided to facilitate resorption of the air within the pleural space.

During the periprocedure and postprocedure activities, it is important to limit all patient activities that may increase intrathoracic pressure and the risk of developing an air leak leading to a pneumothorax. Activities such as coughing, sitting up without assistance, deep breathing, and straining can cause a visceral pleura air leak and the subsequent collapse of the lung.

No chest X-ray is needed immediately after the procedure unless the patient has symptoms related to shortness of breath or is found to have decreasing oxygen saturation. The most important time to protect the puncture site by placing the patient in a puncture-site-down position is the immediate post-biopsy period; a chest X-ray obtained at this time increases the risk of developing a pneumothorax.

The patient should be kept in the puncture-site-down position for 1–2 h; upright expiratory films are obtained at 1 and 2 h postprocedure. If no pneumothorax has developed after 2 h, or if the small initial pneumothorax is unchanged, the patient is allowed to sit up in bed and may move about the room without any type of strenuous activity. A third chest X-ray is obtained 3 h after biopsy; if this image shows no pneumothorax (or no increase in a small pneumothorax), the patient is discharged to home.

Multiple chest X-rays taken an hour apart starting 1 h after the biopsy are useful for pneumothorax surveillance. If an air leak is detected on the first follow-up chest X-ray, oxygen can be applied, the patient is returned to the puncture-site-down position, and aspiration of the pneumothorax is contemplated. The 2-h follow-up will provide a comparison reference to assess whether the air leak has stopped or not. Using this protocol of follow-up, the patients must lie puncture-side-down until they have had no air leakage for an hour. If an interval air leak develops, either invasive treatment is rendered to evacuate the pneumothorax or the patient is returned to the puncture-side-down position, and follow-up is continued.

If the third chest X-ray shows no air leakage, the patient may be discharged. It is important to allow light activity 1 h before the final film is obtained in an attempt to ascertain whether activities similar to the type the patient will be doing at home will cause an air leak. As disheartening as it is to see a pneumothorax develop in the interval between the second and third films, it is extremely important to detect this before the patient is sent home.

Activity Restrictions and Discharge

The procedure should be discussed with the patient in terms of success, complications, and any additional follow-up that will be needed. Optimally, written instructions should be given to the patient along with information outlining the important points of the biopsy procedure (i.e., which lung was biopsied) and whether there was any pneumothorax at the time of discharge. Patient instructions should include guidance about activity (i.e., no straining, lifting, yelling, or other strenuous activity that would increase intrathoracic pressure), diet (no special instructions), and signs/symptoms of developing complications. Patients should limit themselves to only light activity for at least 48–72 h and should be aware that symptoms of shortness of breath or significant hemoptysis (more than a teaspoon full of fresh red blood) signify the need to seek emergency attention. When leaving the hospital the patient should be accompanied by a family member or a friend and should spend the night with someone else nearby.

The emergency contact information should be contained on the discharge instruction sheet so the patient is aware of the appropriate method of seeking emergency care. The discharge instruction sheet should also contain an estimation of the size of the patient's pneumothorax if he or she was discharged with one. The distance from the superiormost portion of the collapsed lung to the thoracic apex may best estimate the size of the pneumothorax.

If the patient is discharged with a pneumothorax, he or she should not travel to high altitudes or fly in a plane for a few days. This will cause pleural stress and may lead to the development of a larger pneumothorax. Obviously the length of time that an individual should avoid high-altitude exposure varies according to the size of the initial pneumothorax. If there is ever a question of reasonable safety, the patient can always return to the Radiology Department for a follow-up X-ray before any travel.

The decision of whether to admit or discharge someone varies from patient to patient and depends on the presence or absence of complications, the severity of any untoward event, the patient's overall health status, the home living situation, and many other factors. The patient's well-being must be considered along with any special circumstances that may influence the discharge and recovery.

Discussion of preliminary cytologic results with the patient is generally not advised because the final histologic diagnosis can vary significantly from the initial reading. Once the pathologist has entered the final diagnosis, however, this may be communicated directly to the patient and must be relayed to the referring clinician for prompt initiation of treatment. It is also important to inform the referring clinician of any complications that occur as well as extenuating circumstances that could have an effect on the patient or the biopsy specimen (i.e., hospital admission, suboptimal needle placement, and so on).

Summary

In general, lung biopsy requires familiarity with the appropriate procedural techniques as well as adequate equipment and preprocedure planning. Potential complications of the procedure must also be considered and appropriate precautions taken in preparation for any untoward events. As important as is the technical strategy for obtaining tissue from the biopsy target, adequate and appropriate communication with the patient is more imperative, and an adequately prepared patient can make the difference between a successful and unsuccessful procedure.

The techniques discussed in this section can provide basic information for the establishment or continuation of a lung biopsy service. Although the lung biopsy process involves many details, patient safety, procedural efficacy, and diagnostic accuracy are all of paramount importance and must be appropriately balanced if a successful lung biopsy program is to be maintained.

3 ARTHROGRAPHY

Arthrography has been performed since the 1930s and is a technically straightforward procedure that can be safely performed on nearly all patients. It has been shown to have a high level of diagnostic accuracy and is a widely accepted routine diagnostic procedure. Although technical improvements in the latter part of the 20th century (i.e., submillimeter focal spot X-ray tubes and improved image intensifiers) have significantly improved the quality and diagnostic consistency of arthrography, much of its utility has been replaced by MRI. Nevertheless, the technique of arthrography remains important not only for conventional radiographic exams but also for widespread practice of magnetic resonance arthrography.

Arthrography Equipment

The equipment set used for joint intervention is very similar for most of the joints commonly subjected to arthrography. An example of the typical arthrogram set is presented below. Alterations in the composition of the set may be necessary according to the specific needs of the institutions where these procedures are performed. There are also many commercially available arthrogram sets that provide prepackaged arthrography materials.

Arthrography Equipment Set

–One 10-mL syringe (Luer-Lok®)
–One 20-mL syringe (Luer-Lok)

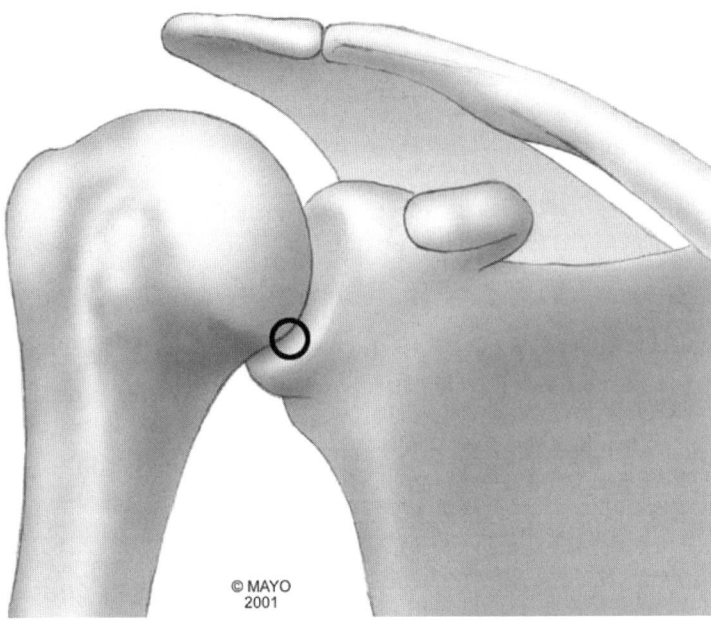

© MAYO
2001

Fig. 11. Shoulder arthrogram. Image taken in a supine position with the shoulder in external rotation. The circle indicates the needle target position.

−One 5-mL syringe (Luer-Lok)

−One 25g 5/8-inch needle

−One 20-g × 1.5-inch needle

−One 22-g × 1.5-inch needle

−One 20-g × 3.5-inch spinal needle

−One 22-g × 3.5-inch spinal needle

−Sterile drape (cloth or paper) with 5-cm round hole

−5 mL 1% lidocaine solution

−Sterile plastic tubing

−10 mL sterile saline (no preservative)

−Povidone-iodine solution for skin preparation

−Forceps (plastic or metallic)

−Gauze sponges (at least five 4 × 3-inch sponges)

−Sterile surgical gloves

−Diatrizoate meglumine 60% (Hypaque® 60%) or similar type of meglumine iodinated contrast

Complications

As in any procedure in which a needle transgresses the skin, there are risks of bleeding, infection, and injury to an underlying structure. Provided there is adequate antiseptic skin preparation, infection is a rare complication, with a reported incidence as low as 1 in 25,000. In patients without known coagulopathies, the risk of hemorrhage is also extremely low.

One of the more common complications of arthrography is allergic reaction to the injected contrast. The risk is approximately 1 in 1000 for mild allergic reaction after intraarticular contrast injection. Most of these reactions will occur within 20 min after the injection of contrast.

An unusual complication specifically related to arthrography is that of a sterile synovial effusion. This occurs in approximately 1 in 1000 patients and is manifested by pain and stiffness of the affected joint. The effusion usually develops within the first 8–12 h after the examination, and subsequent aspiration will not only alleviate the patient's symptoms but will also document the absence of bacteriologic contamination. The etiology of this complication is thought to be a chemical or allergic synovitis. Joint effusion has also been reported in patients who participate in vigorous or athletic activities with 1–2 days after the arthrogram.

Shoulder Arthrography (Single Contrast)

1. Complete radiographic exam of the shoulder should be obtained before the arthrogram to evaluate any bony abnormalities.

2. The patient is placed supine on the fluoroscopic table, and the shoulder of interest is placed flat against the table. The arm should be placed in slight external rotation, and the contralateral shoulder should be minimally elevated (by using towels, sheets, or iv bags placed under the scapula) to facilitate appropriate positioning. Slight anterior angulation of the glenoid fossa with minimal glenohumeral overlap (See Fig. 11) will allow the needle to pass freely into the joint without penetrating the glenoid labrum.

3. After application of the antiseptic iodine solution and using sterile technique, the local anesthetic needle (a 22-g 1½-inch needle) is placed over the appropriate target position (Fig. 11) via fluoroscopic guidance. Subsequently, 2–3 mL of 1% lidocaine is infiltrated intradermally and into the deeper soft tissues of the shoulder.

4. Using fluoroscopic guidance, a 22-g spinal needle is inserted into the glenohumeral joint. The needle should be advanced

assessment can be documented either as a formal consultation or in an assessment form. Consent to perform the procedure should also be obtained. This consent can either be verbal or written depending on the institutional policy for obtaining procedural consent.

Preprocedure Orders

After obtaining the appropriate history, clinical information, and consent for the procedure, preprocedure orders should be furnished if there is an opportunity to do so. An example of these orders is as follows:

1. Allergies: _____
2. npo except for medications
3. Start saline lock
4. Patient may take own medications as follows: _____
5. Preprocedure antibiotics: _____
6. Preprocedure medications: _____
7. Other orders: _____
8. Contact vascular/interventional radiology at _____ for questions or orders.

Presenting the Case to the Attending Physician

Present the case in a concise and objective manner.

1. Procedure requested, requesting service.
2. Patient's age, symptoms, pertinent previous interventions/ surgery, allergies.
3. Pulse evaluation.
4. Relevant laboratory results.
5. Show pertinent imaging studies.

After discussion of the case, decide about the access site, contrast type, catheters and wires to be used.

Talking to Ancillary Personnel

The nurse and the radiologic technologist should be informed of the planned access site, catheters, and wires you will use, and the type of contrast with which to load the power injector and the flush line. All patients should have an iv access.

When performing a lower extremity angiogram, let the technologist know what type of image acquisition technique will be used:

- DSA (digital subtracted image)
- DA (digital nonsubtracted)
- Cut films (rapid sequence of films using 14 × 14 film)
- Road mapping (stored image with superimposed live fluoroscopy)
- Automated peripheral subtracted angiography (i.e., Perivision).

Special Problems

Prophylactic antibiotics decrease the incidence of postprocedure infection/bacteremia in certain procedures. Routine indications include biliary and genitourinary interventions, chemoembolization, tumor ablation, dialysis graft angioplasty and TIPSS. Some of the commonly used regimens are as follows:

- *Cefazolin (Ancef®),* 1 g iv
- *Piperacillin sodium* and *tazobactam sodium (Zosyn®),* 3.375 g iv
- *Ampicillin sodium/sulbactam sodium (Unasyn®),* 1.5–3.0 g iv
- *Vancomycin* 1 g iv (for penicillin allergy).

Diabetic patients should reduce their insulin dosage on the procedure day or hold the oral hypoglycemic.

Patients with a significant history of contrast allergy require premedication. Suggested regimens include:

- Methylprednisolone (Medrol®) 32 mg po 12 h and 2 h before exam *or*
- Prednisone 40 mg po 12–18 h and 2 h before exam
- Diphenhydramine (Benadryl®) 50 mg po or im 1 h before exam (optional).

2 HARDWARE

Needles and Introducer Sets

A large variety of hardware is used in vascular and interventional radiology procedures, and an exhaustive list of these various components would be beyond the scope of this section. There are many different ways of performing similar procedures, and the various tools used primarily reflect the personal preferences of the operator. The list of hardware included in this chapter illustrates some of the most commonly used devices.

There are also many different types of vascular access needles. The needles are sized by gage, with the higher numbers indicating smaller needle diameters (the higher the gage number, the smaller the diameter of the needle).

For arterial punctures, the following needles may be used:

- Hollow needle with sharp stylet (Potts-type needle) *(Fig. 14)*
- Alternatively, there are hollow needles without the stylet *(Fig. 15)*
- A micropuncture set consists of a smaller and less traumatic needle (21-g, 7 cm), 0.018-inch guidewire (40 cm), and 4-Fr coaxial catheter. It is commonly used in pediatric patients, difficult femoral artery punctures, and brachial artery punctures. Micropuncture sets may also be used for jugular vein access and dialysis fistulograms *(Fig. 16).*

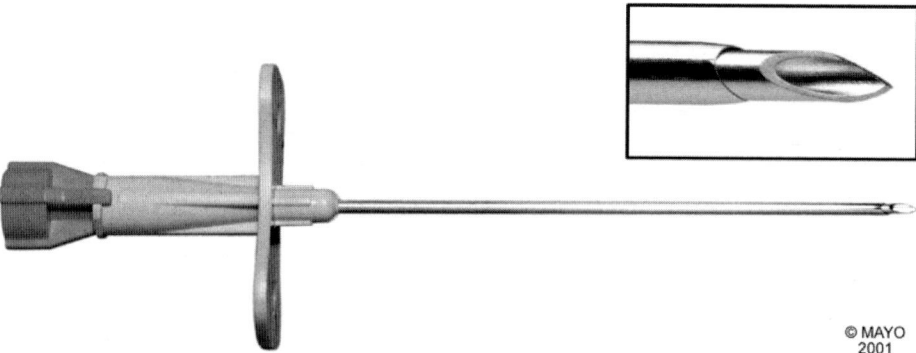

Fig. 14. Potts needle with stylet.

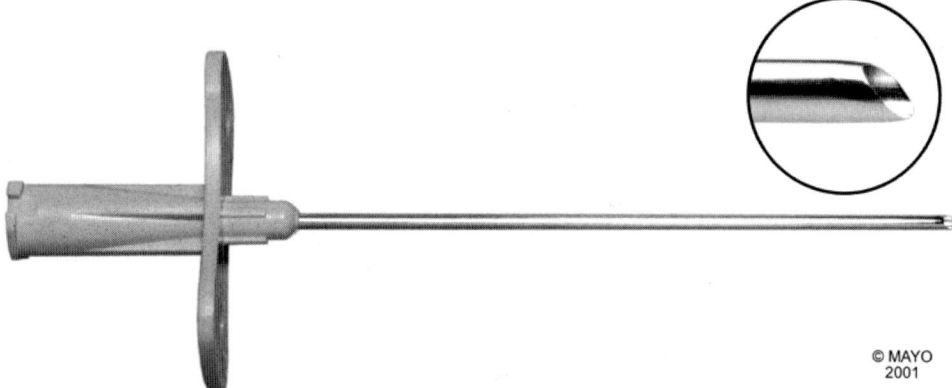

Fig. 15. Potts needle without stylet.

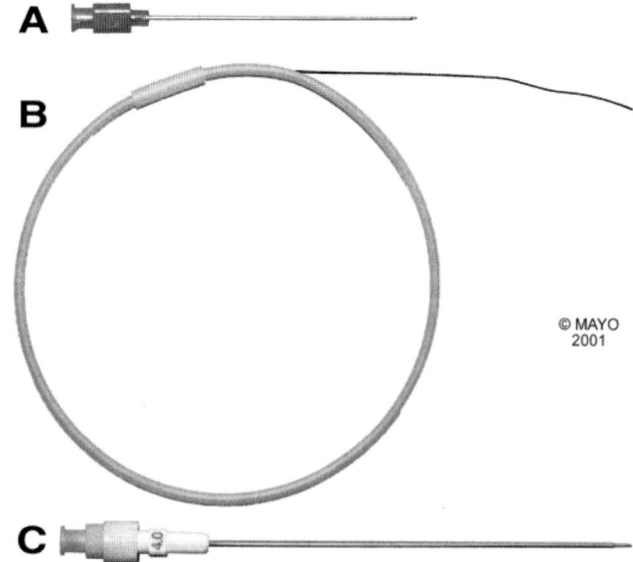

Fig. 16. Micropuncture set. The set consists of a 7-cm, 21-g needle (**A**), a 40-cm 0.018-inch guidewire (**B**), and a 4-Fr coaxial catheter (**C**).

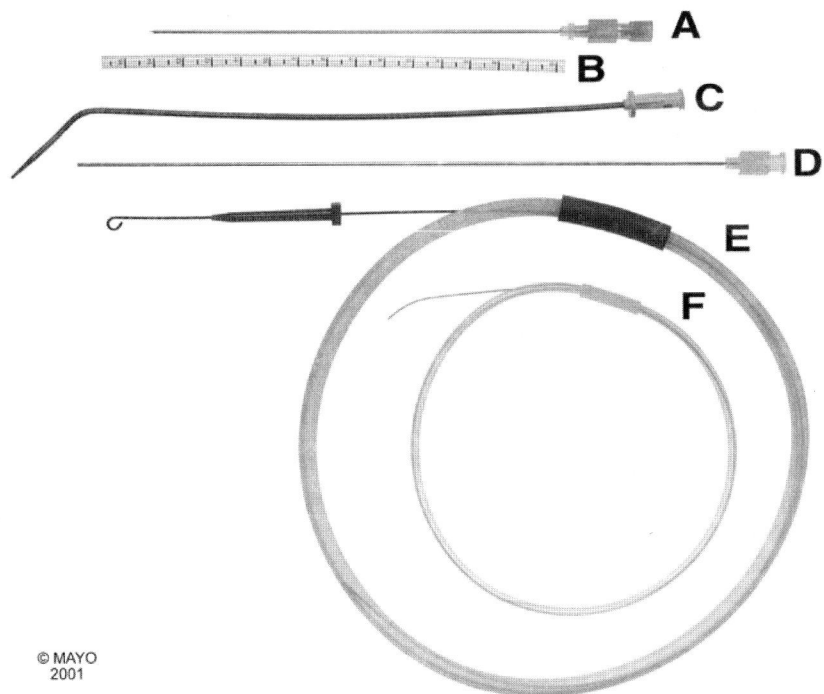

Fig. 17. Cope set. The Cope set consists of a 21-g needle (**A**), a ruler (**B**), a 6.3-Fr dilator (**C**), a metal stiffer for the dilator (**D**), a 0.035-inch guidewire (**E**), and a 0.018-inch guidewire (**F**).

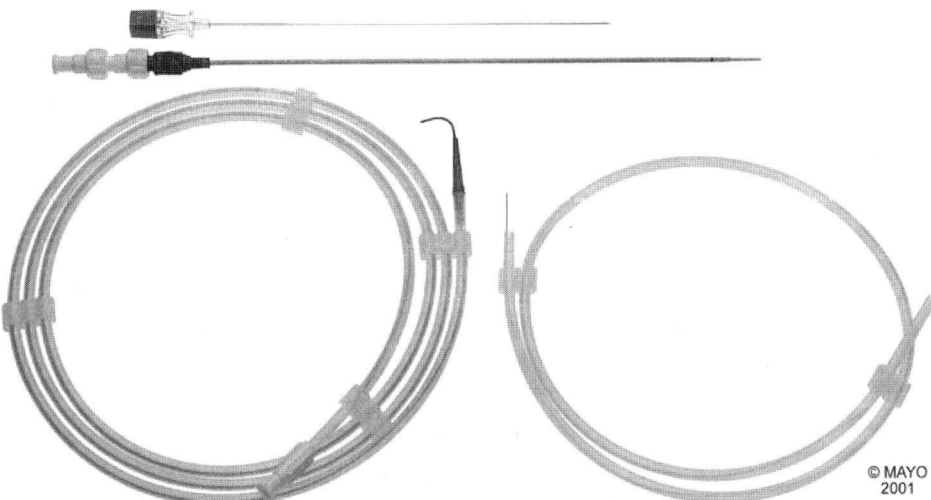

Fig. 18. Accustick set. The Accustick set consists of a 21-g, 15-cm needle (**A**), a 4.5-Fr dilator (**B**), a 0.035-inch guidewire (**C**), and a 0.018-inch guidewire (**D**).

For biliary and genitourinary interventions:

–Chiba needle: 22-g (20 cm), 0.018-inch guidewire *(Fig. 1C)*

–Cope set: 21-g (15 cm), 0.018 and 0.035-inch guidewire, 6.3-Fr dilator *(Fig. 17)*

–Accustick set: 21-g (15 cm), 0.018 and 0.035-inch guidewires, 4.5-Fr dilator *(Fig. 18)*.

For venous puncture:

–18-g, 5-cm hollow needle

–Majestic needle *(Fig. 19)*

–Potts needle.

Dilators/Sheaths

Vascular dilators are used to create a less traumatic track in the tissues before insertion of a catheter or sheath. The dilators

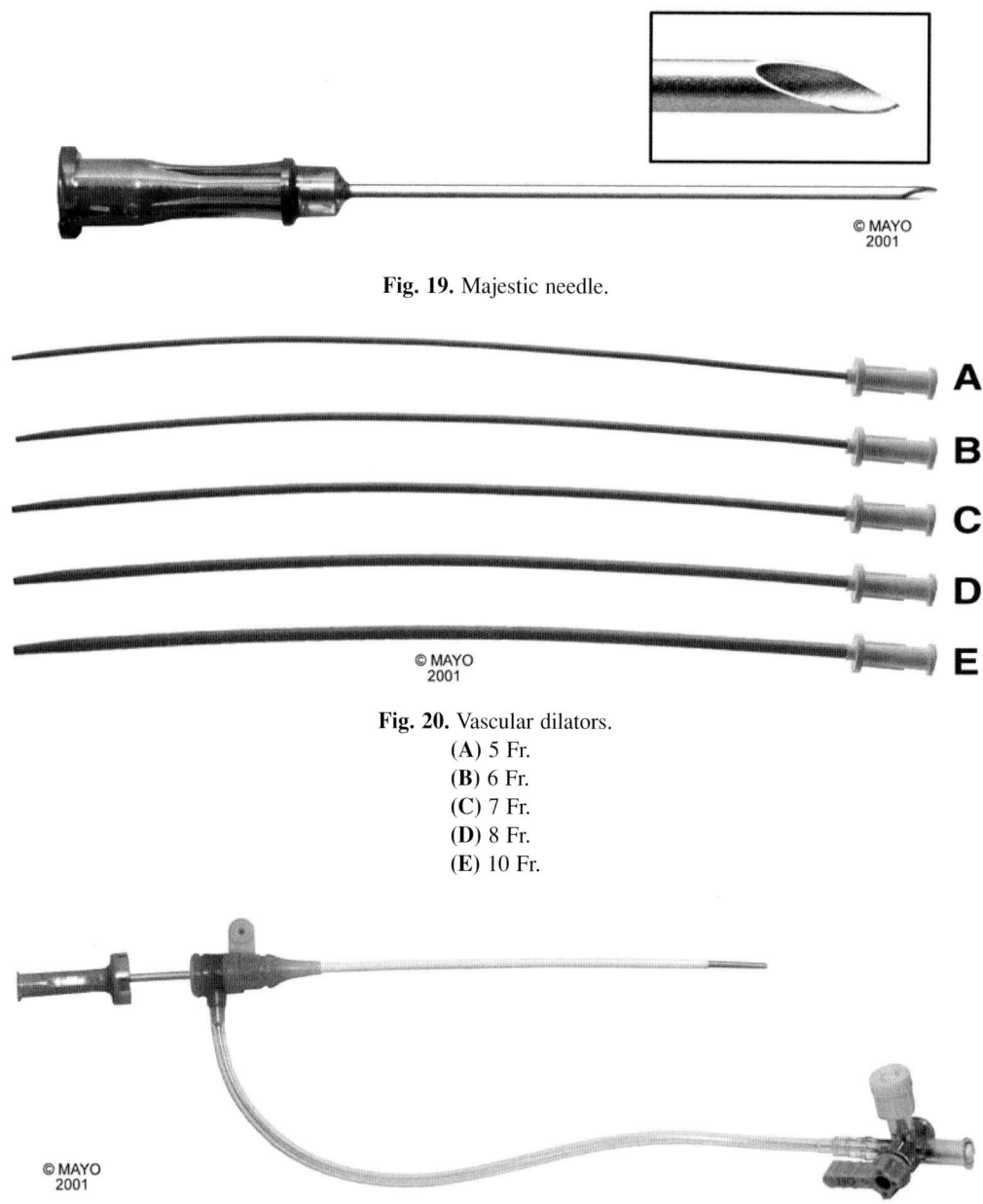

Fig. 19. Majestic needle.

Fig. 20. Vascular dilators.
(**A**) 5 Fr.
(**B**) 6 Fr.
(**C**) 7 Fr.
(**D**) 8 Fr.
(**E**) 10 Fr.

Fig. 21. Vascular introducer sheath (with vascular dilator in place through the outer cannula).

have a tapered end and are available from 4 to 24 Fr (outer diameter [OD]) *(Fig. 20)*. Introducer sheaths in angiography are used if multiple catheter exchanges are expected or if bleeding develops at the puncture site. Introducer sheaths are also widely used for access in nonvascular interventions and drainage of fluid collections. The introducer set consists of a dilator and sheath system with a side port flush line *(Fig. 21)*. They are available in 4–14 Fr (inner diameter [ID]), have lengths ranging from 10 to 90 cm, and can have a radiopaque tip. Long sheaths are used for renal artery stent placement, contralateral iliac artery angioplasty/stent placement, and some nonvascular procedures.

One special type of sheath is the Peel-Away-Sheath. It has a coaxial system with a dilator and an outer sheath that may be peeled away after insertion of a catheter through the inner portion of the sheath. After the outer sheath is peeled away, it is of no use and is discarded. Jugular vein access, biliary/genitourinary interventions, and gastrostomy tube placement are some of the common instances in which the Peel-Away-Sheath is used (it is available in sizes ranging from 7 to 22 Fr) *(Fig. 22)*.

Guidewires

Guidewires are used to introduce safely and select the positioning of catheters. Their structure consists of a central stiff inner

a. Bile leak: contrast extravasation
b. Obstruction (periampullary or cholangiocarcinoma): dilatation of bile ducts proximal to the obstructing lesion
c. Sclerosing cholangitis: stenosis, dilatation (string of beads), and diverticula
I. Percutaneous nephrostomy tube placement
  1. Indications
    a. Hydronephrosis
    b. Pyonephrosis
    c. Therapeutic: stone removal, stent placement
  2. Complications

a. Hematuria: arteriovenous or arteriocaliceal fistula, pseudoaneurysm
b. Infection
c. Urinoma
d. Pneumothorax/empyema
  3. Contraindications
    a. Uncorrectable coagulopathy
  4. Differential diagnosis
    a. Hydronephrosis
    b. Filling defects: stones, blood clot, tumor, gas bubble, fungus ball

7 VASCULAR ANATOMY

The proficient performance of common vascular and non-vascular procedures requires sound fundamental knowledge of the anatomy involved in the particular procedure. Although exhaustive anatomic detail is usually not necessary, a solid base of anatomic knowledge will facilitate consistent procedural success and will provide confidence for less experienced individuals. The following illustrations (Figs. 41–58, pp. 69–84) are designed to illustrate the basic anatomy of various portions of the vascular system and of various organs in order to provide a quick reference and brief anatomic review. These figures are intended to illustrate the anatomy most commonly encountered in a typical practice of vascular and interventional radiology.

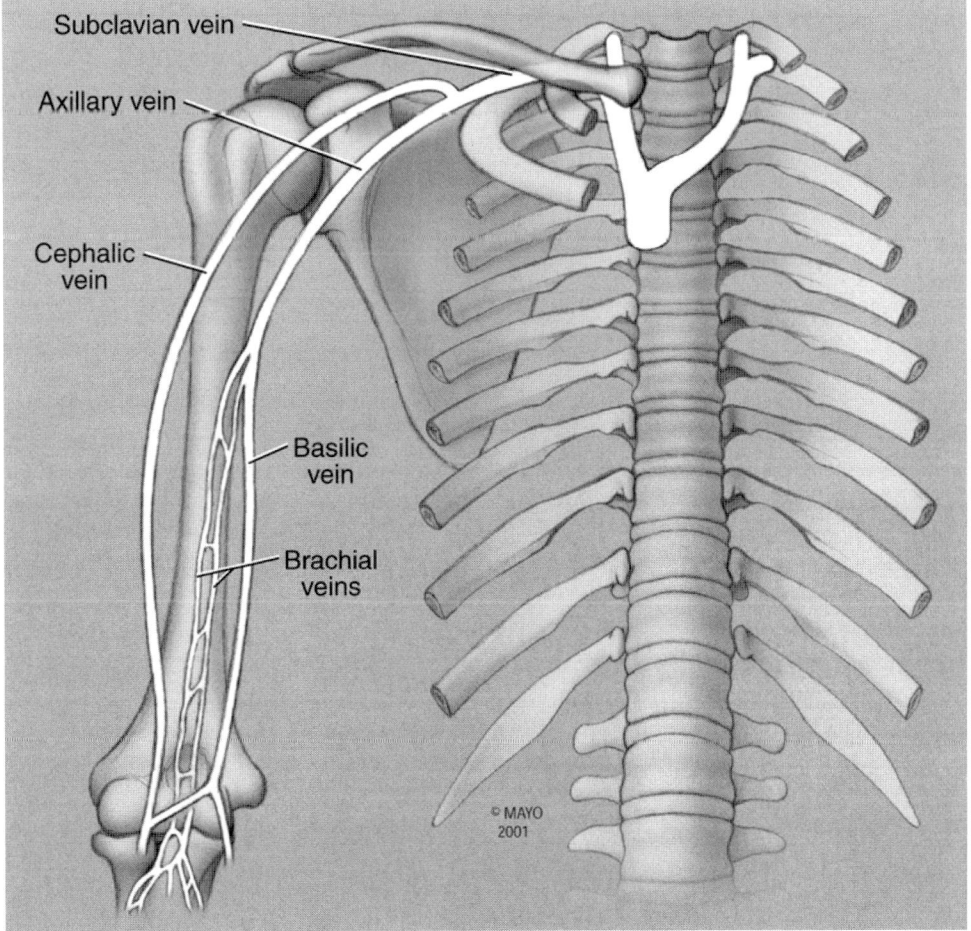

Fig. 41. Upper extremity veins.

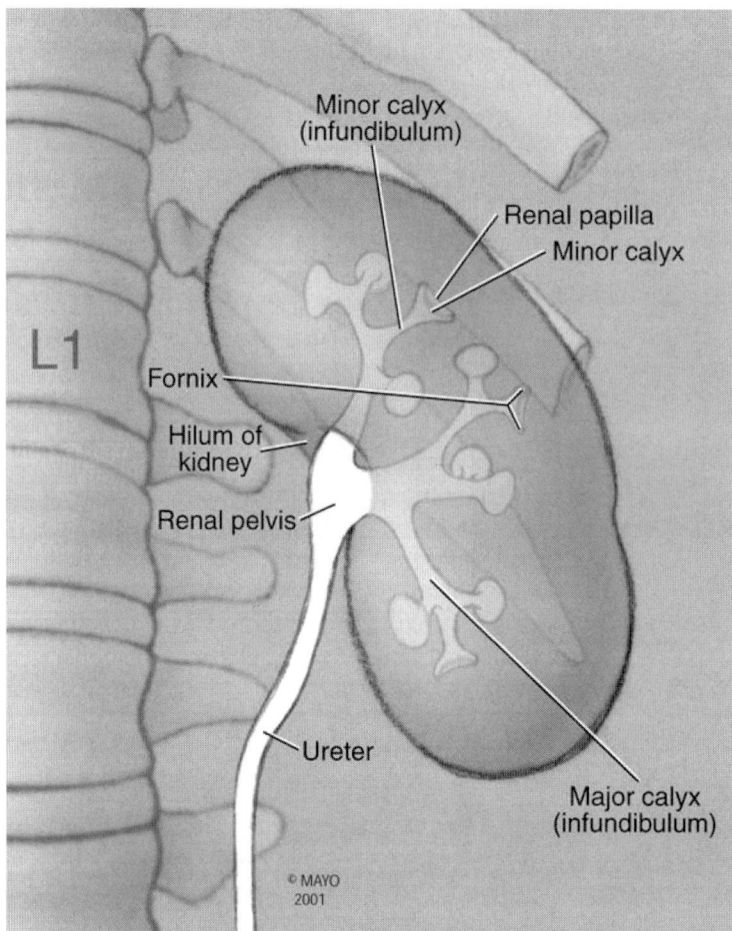

Fig. 42. Renal collecting system anatomy.

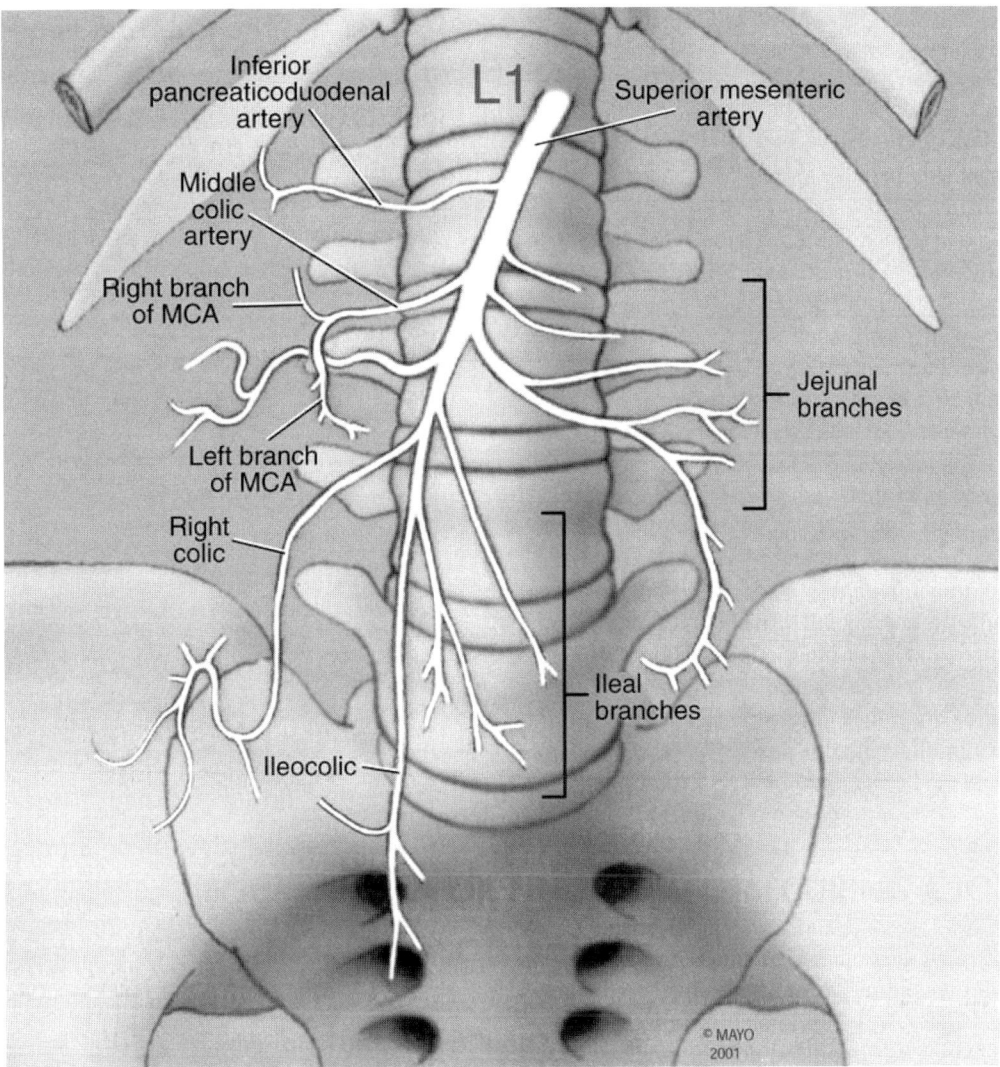

Fig. 43. Superior mesenteric artery. MCA, middle colic artery.

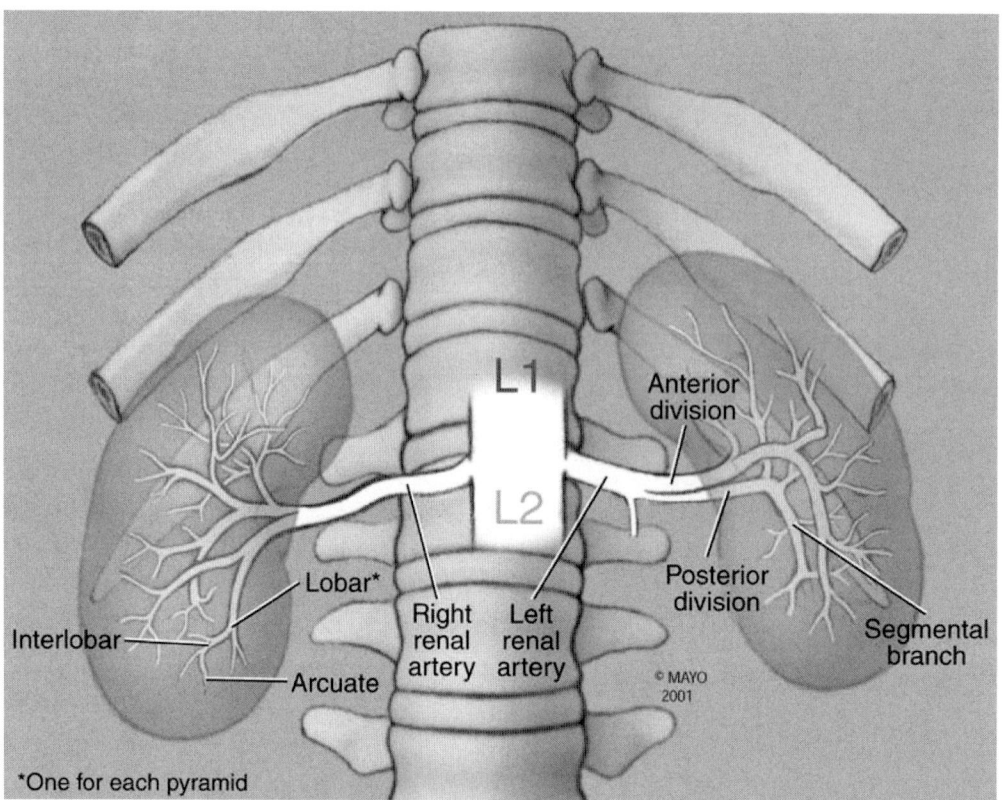

Fig. 44. Renal arteries.

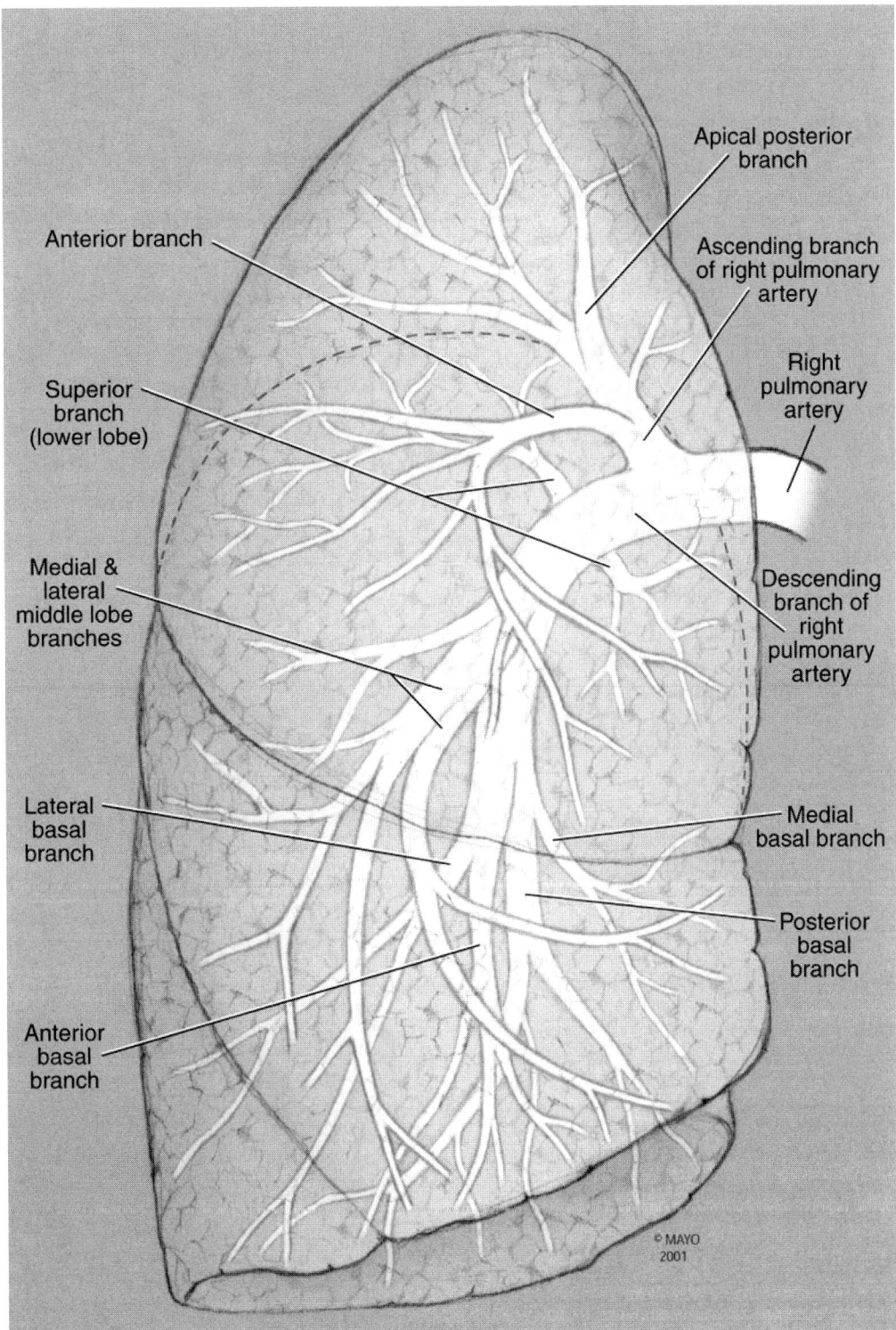

Fig. 45. Right pulmonary arteries.

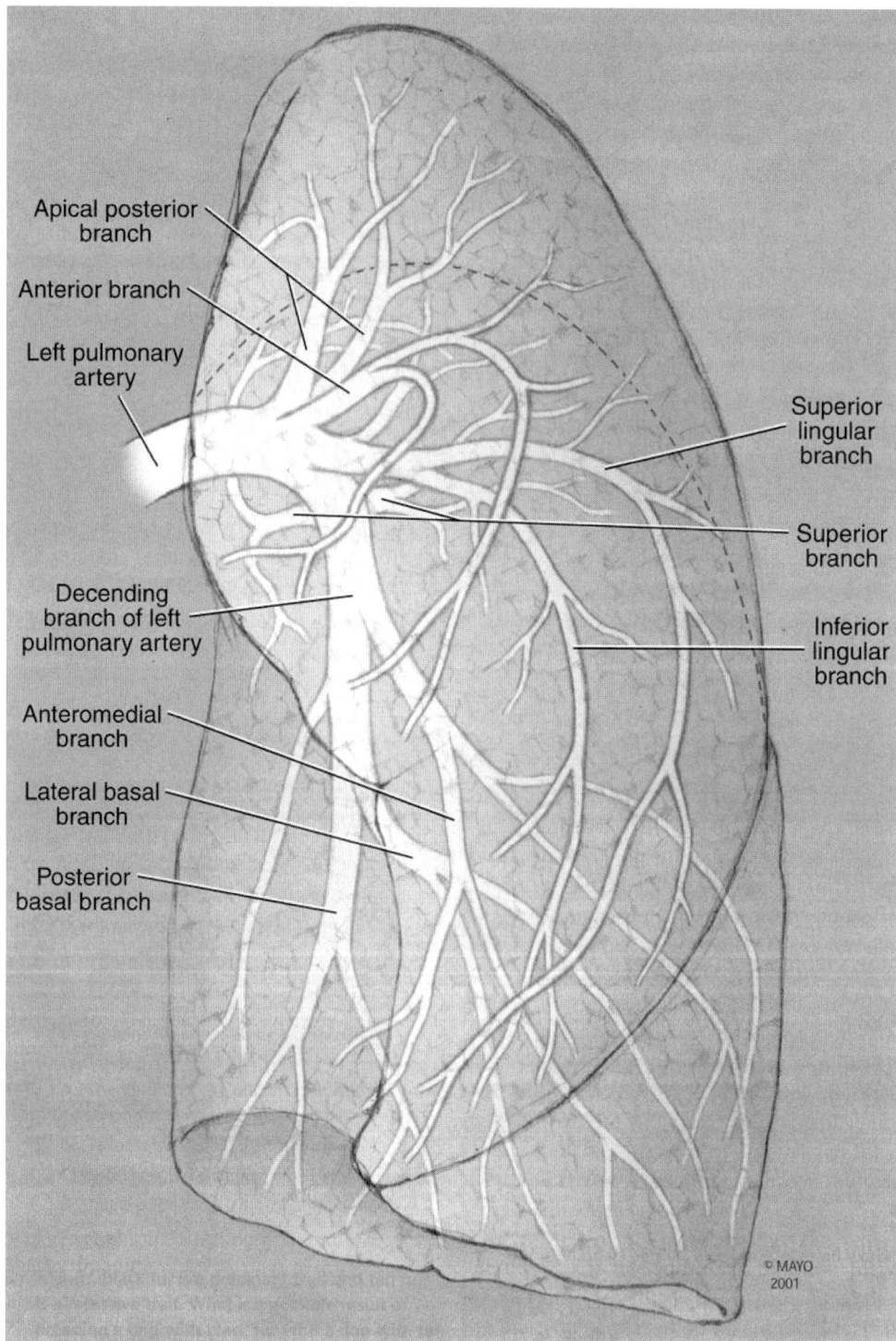

Apical posterior branch

Anterior branch

Left pulmonary artery

Superior lingular branch

Superior branch

Decending branch of left pulmonary artery

Inferior lingular branch

Anteromedial branch

Lateral basal branch

Posterior basal branch

© MAYO 2001

Fig. 46. Left pulmonary arteries.

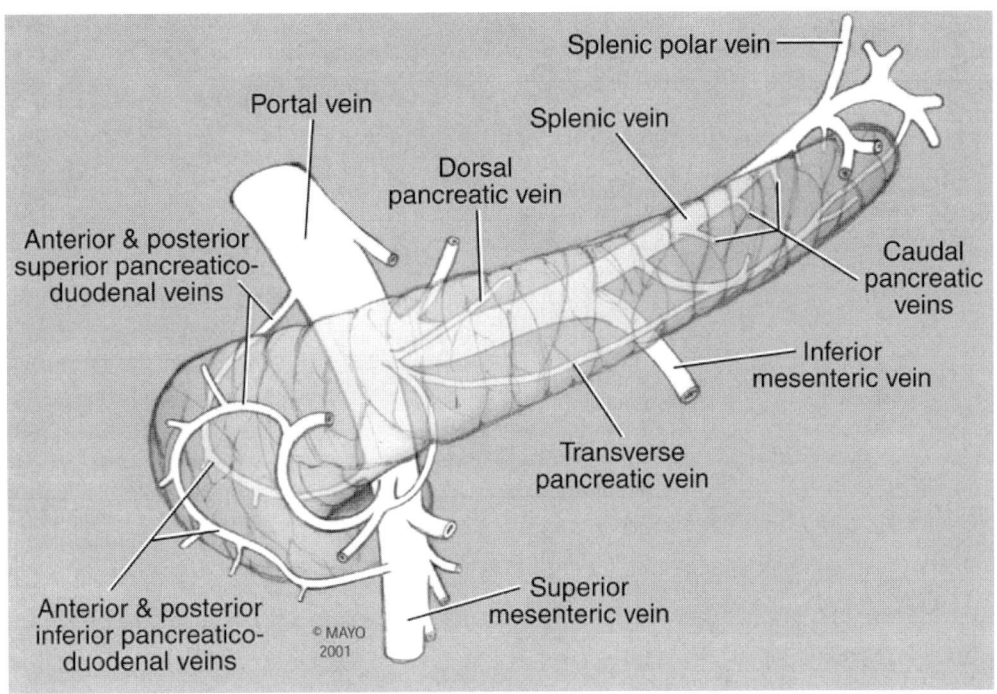

Fig. 47. Peripancreatic portal venous circulation.

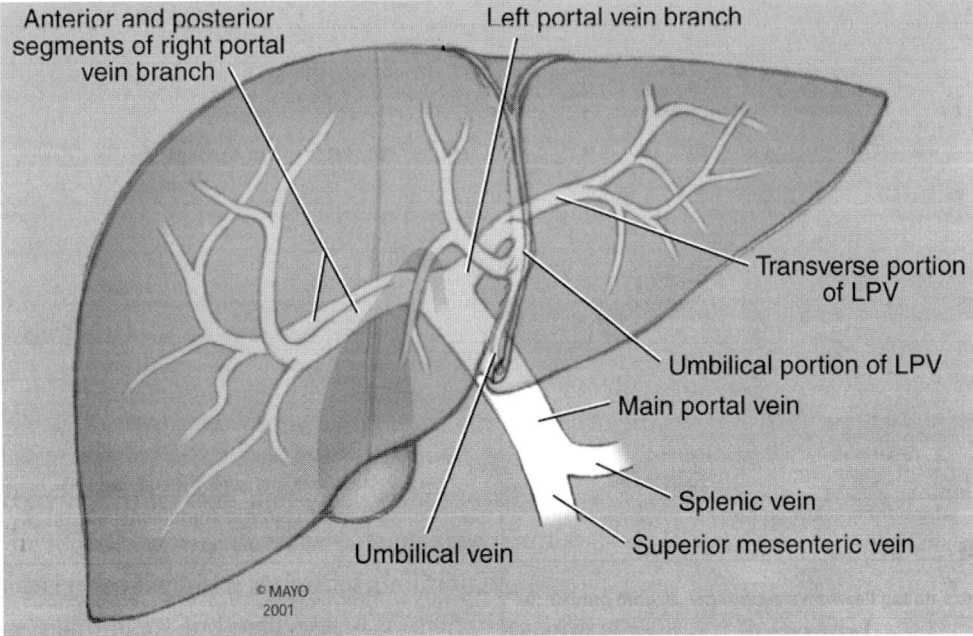

Fig. 48. Portal venous circulation. LPV, left portal vein.

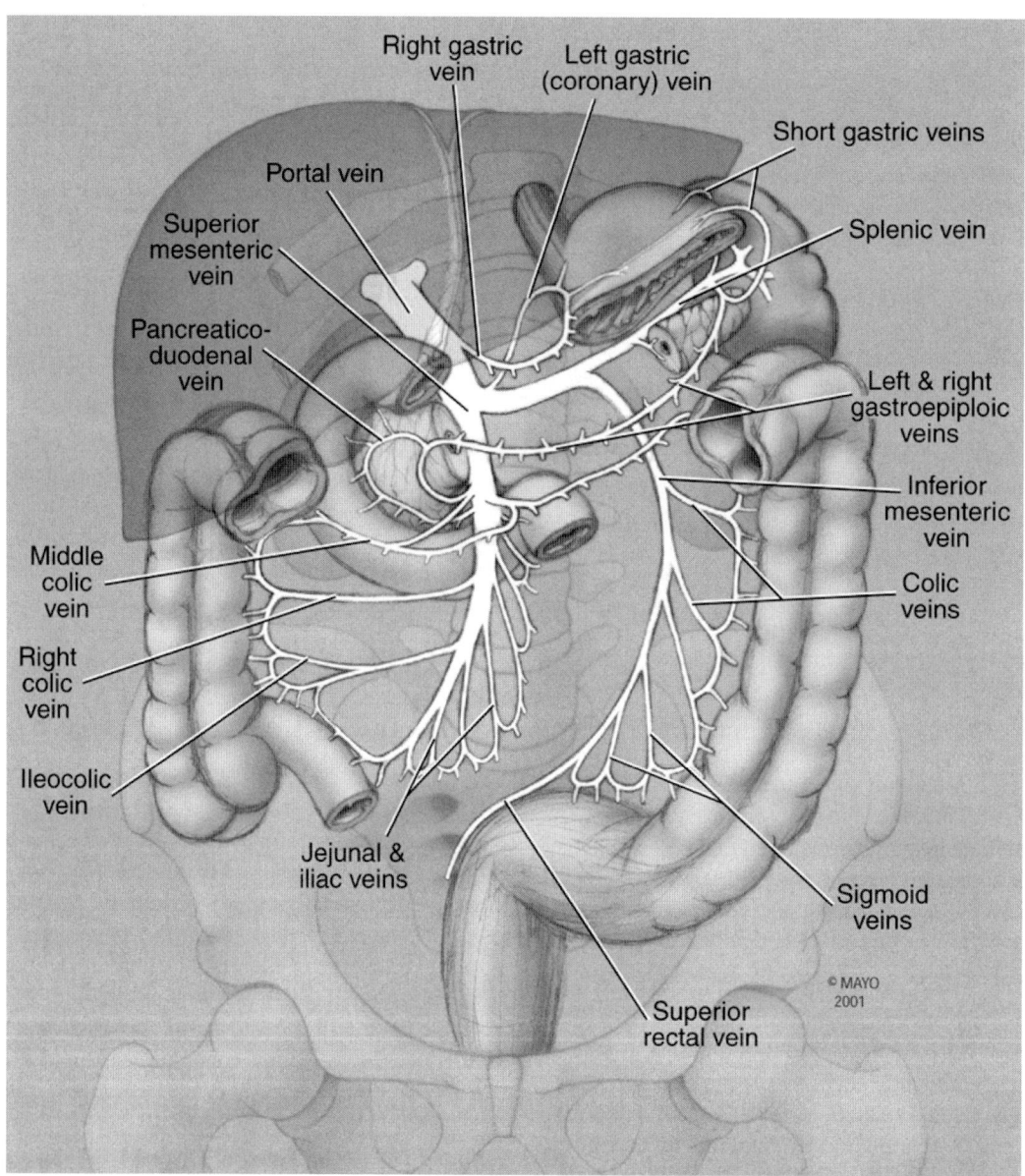

Fig. 49. Portal venous system.

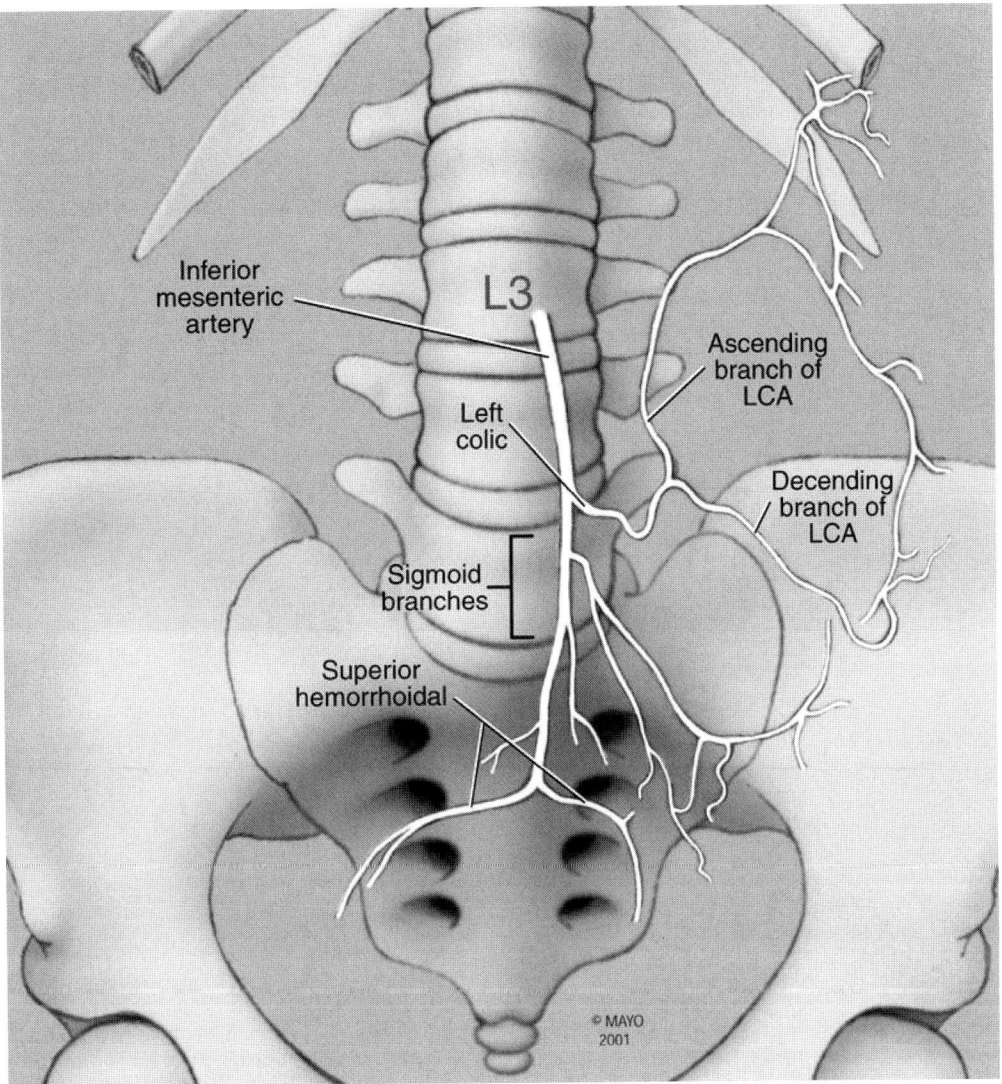

Fig. 50. Inferior mesenteric artery. LCA, Left colic artery.

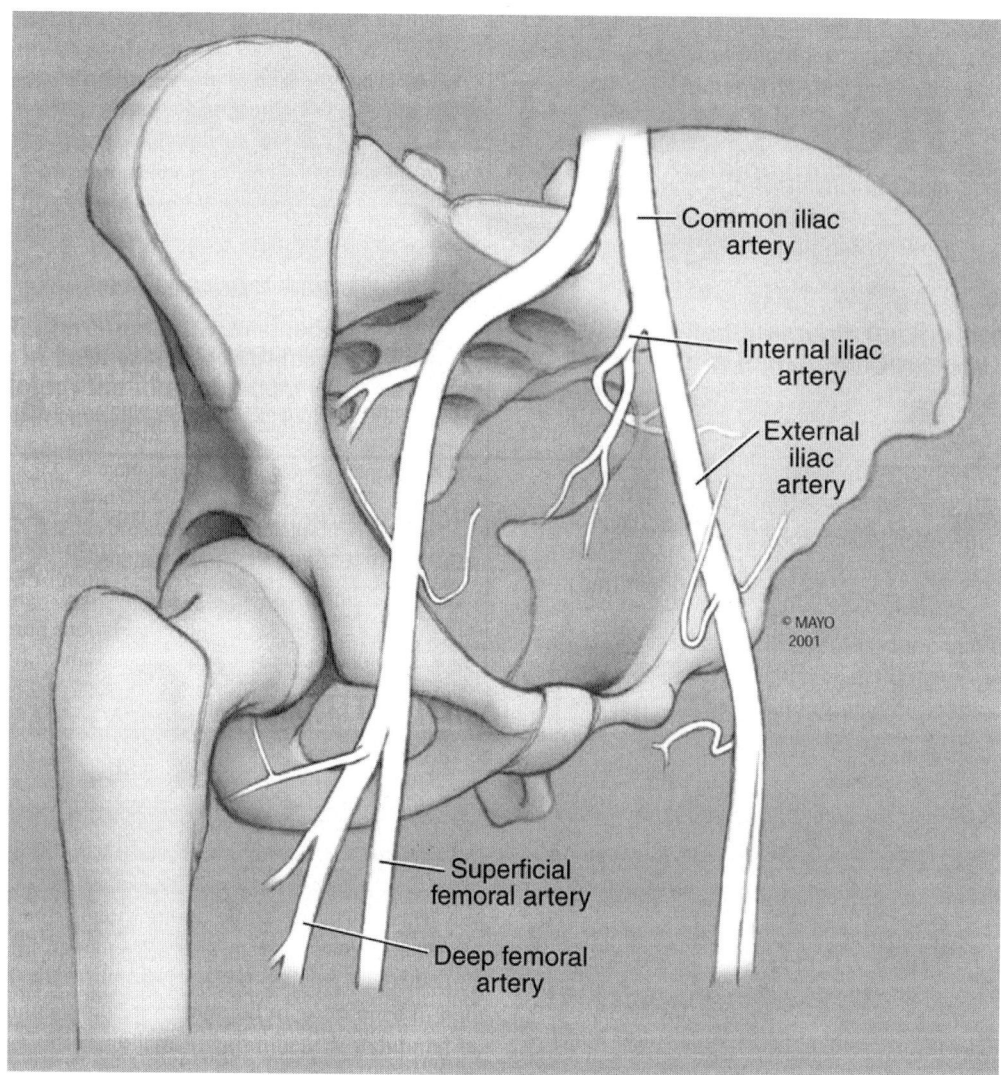

Fig. 51. Iliac arteries (oblique view).

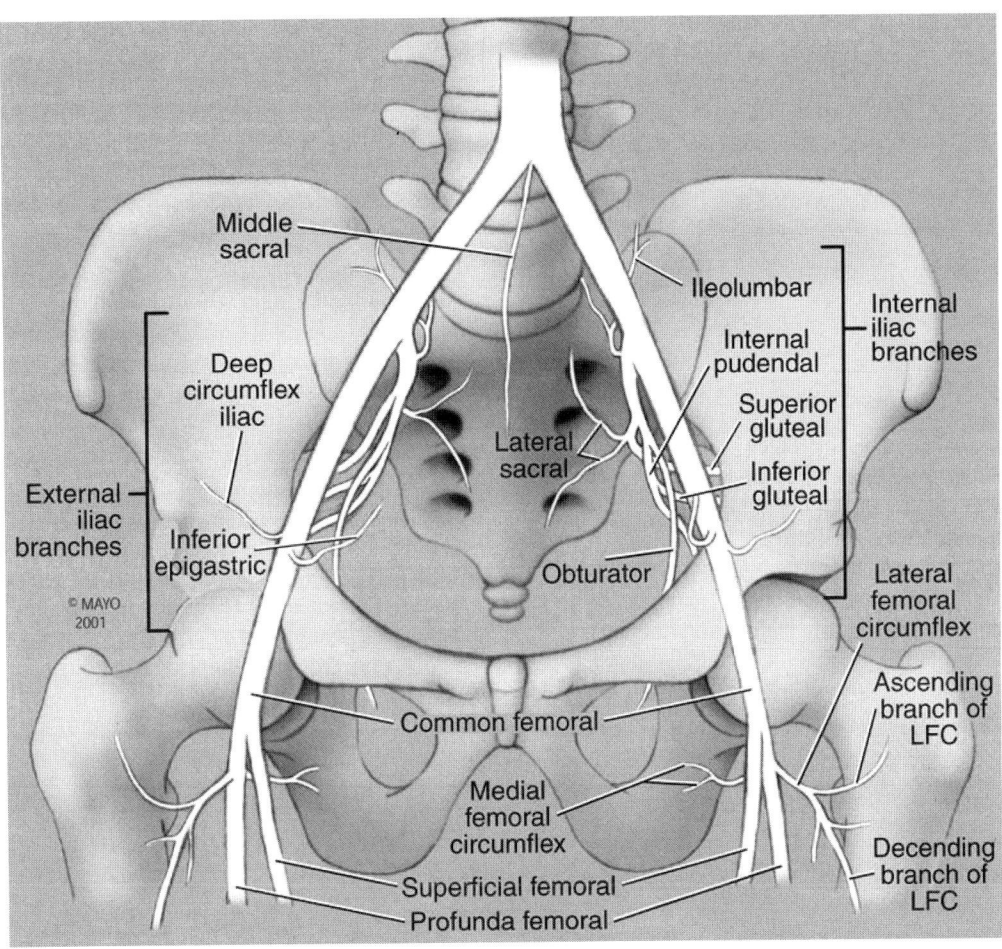

Fig. 52. Iliac arterial circulation. LFC, lateral femoral circumflex.

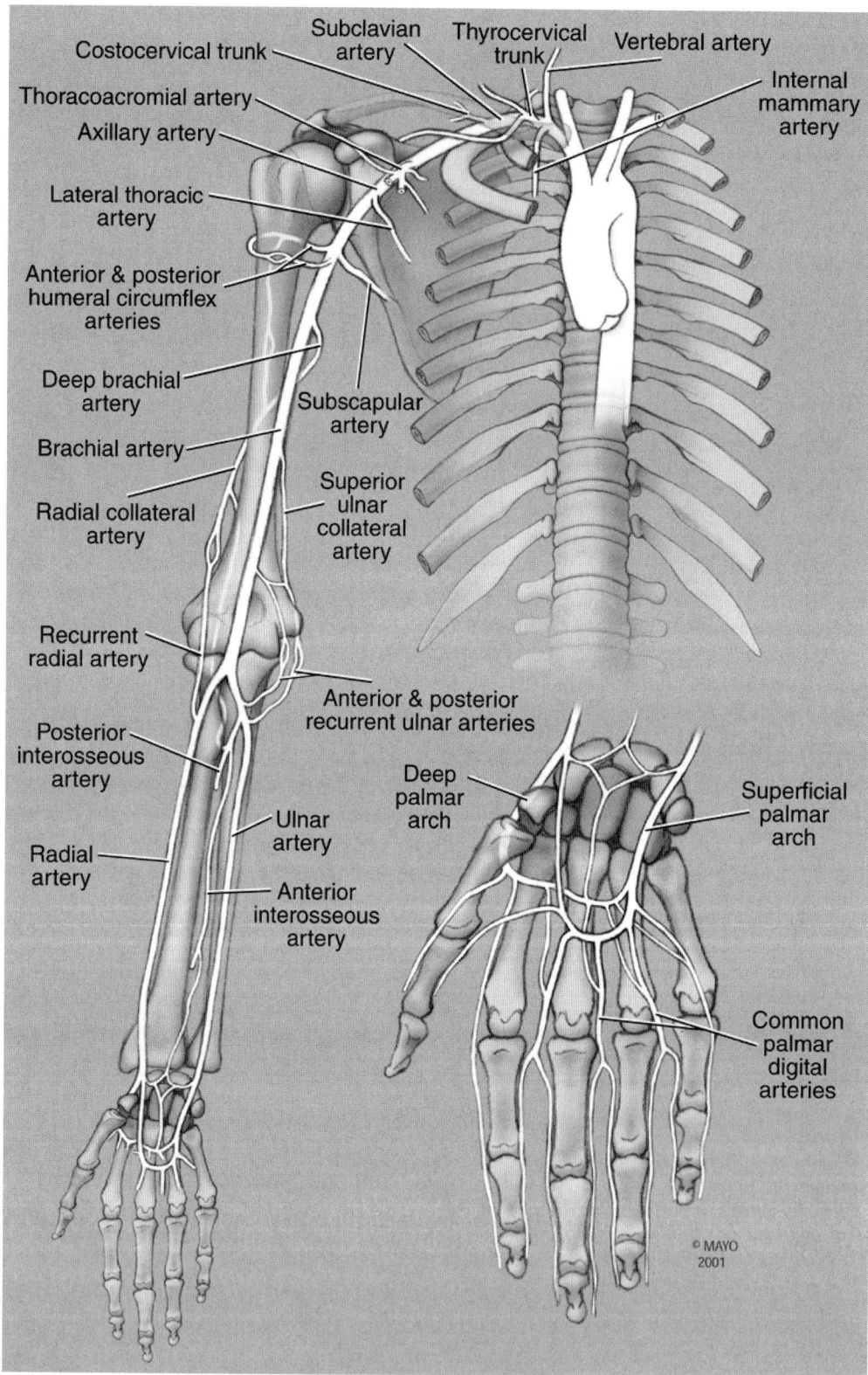

Fig. 53. Upper extremity arteries.

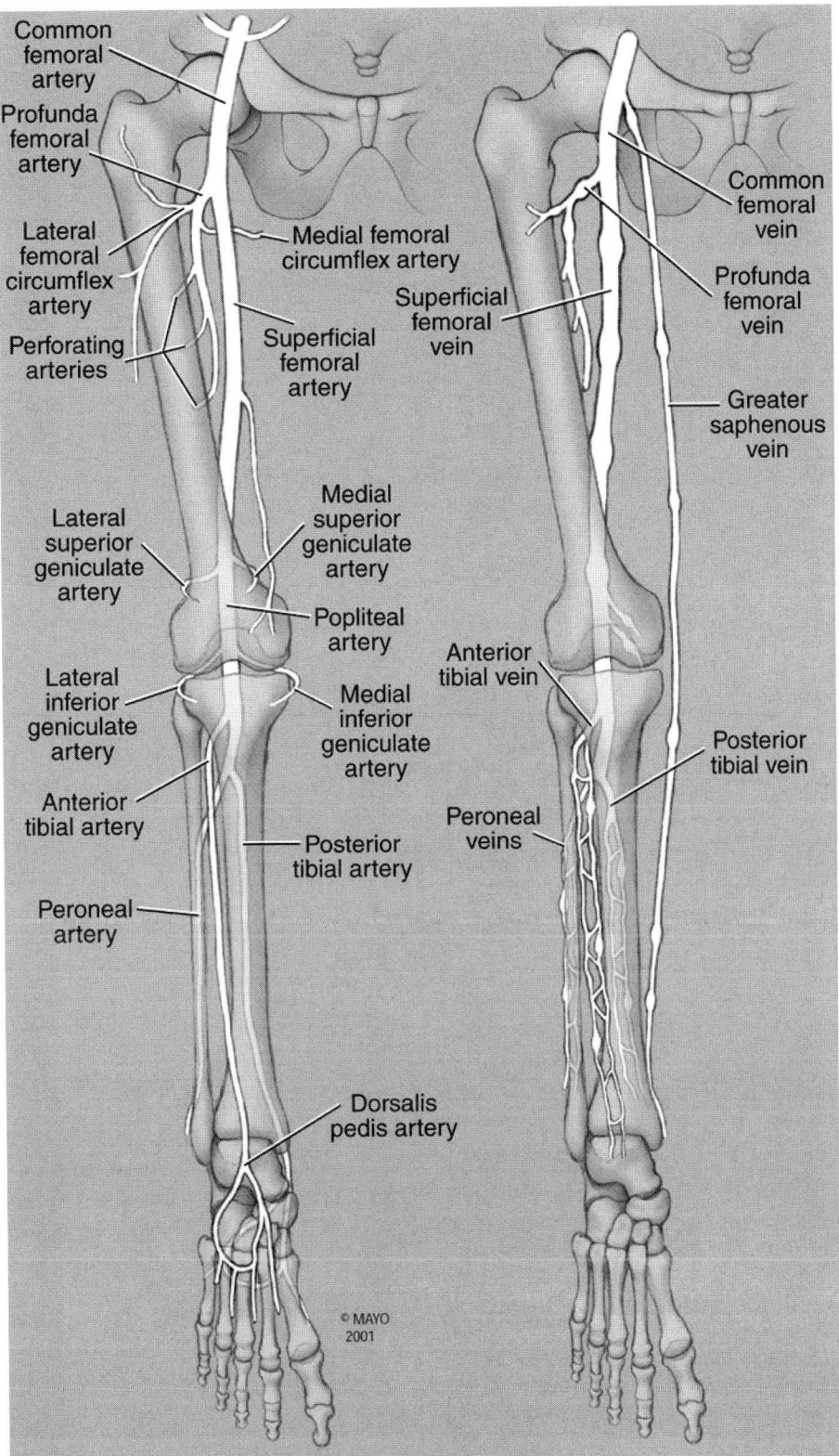

Fig. 54. Lower extremity arteries.

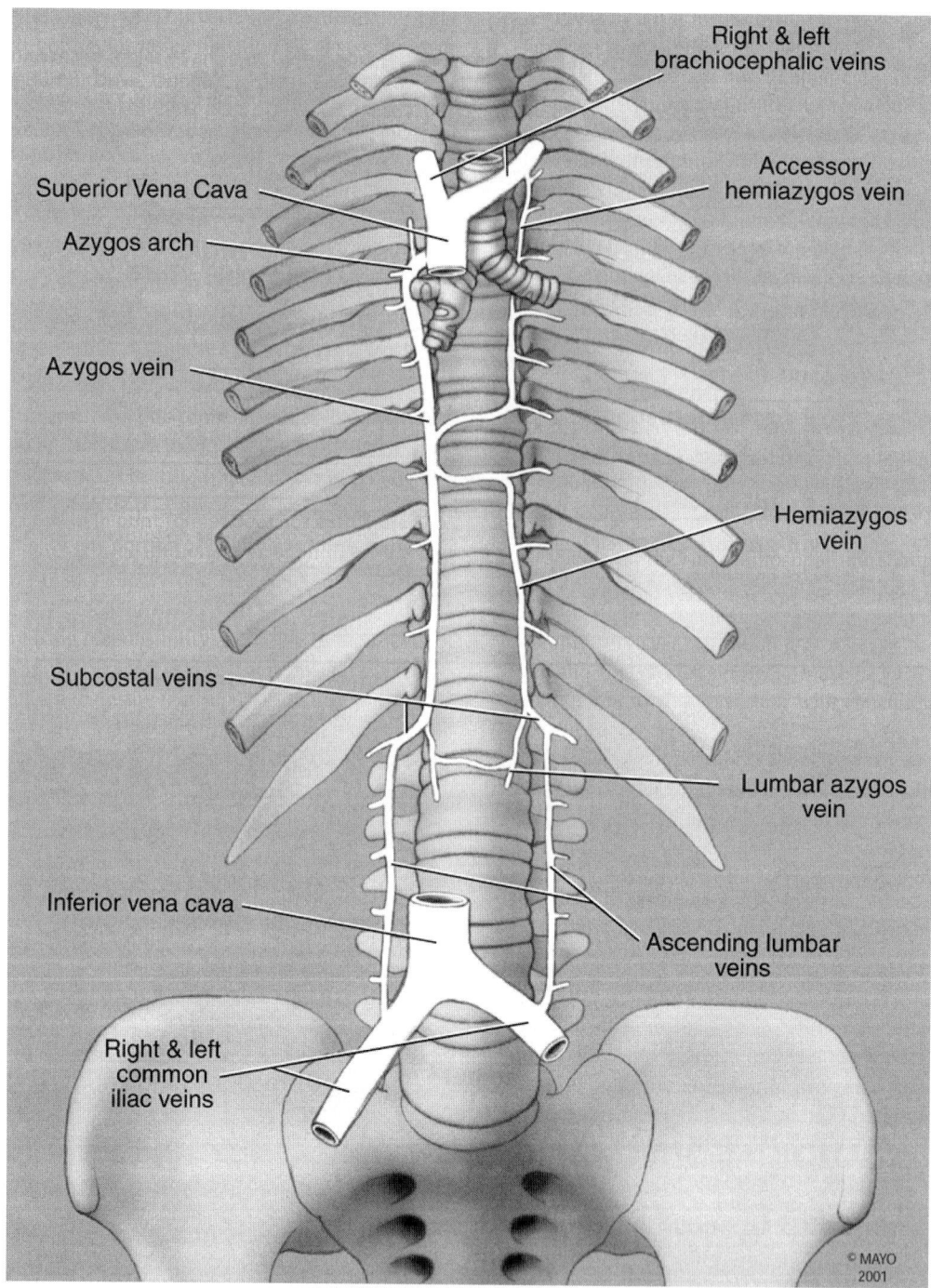

Fig. 55. Azygous venous system.

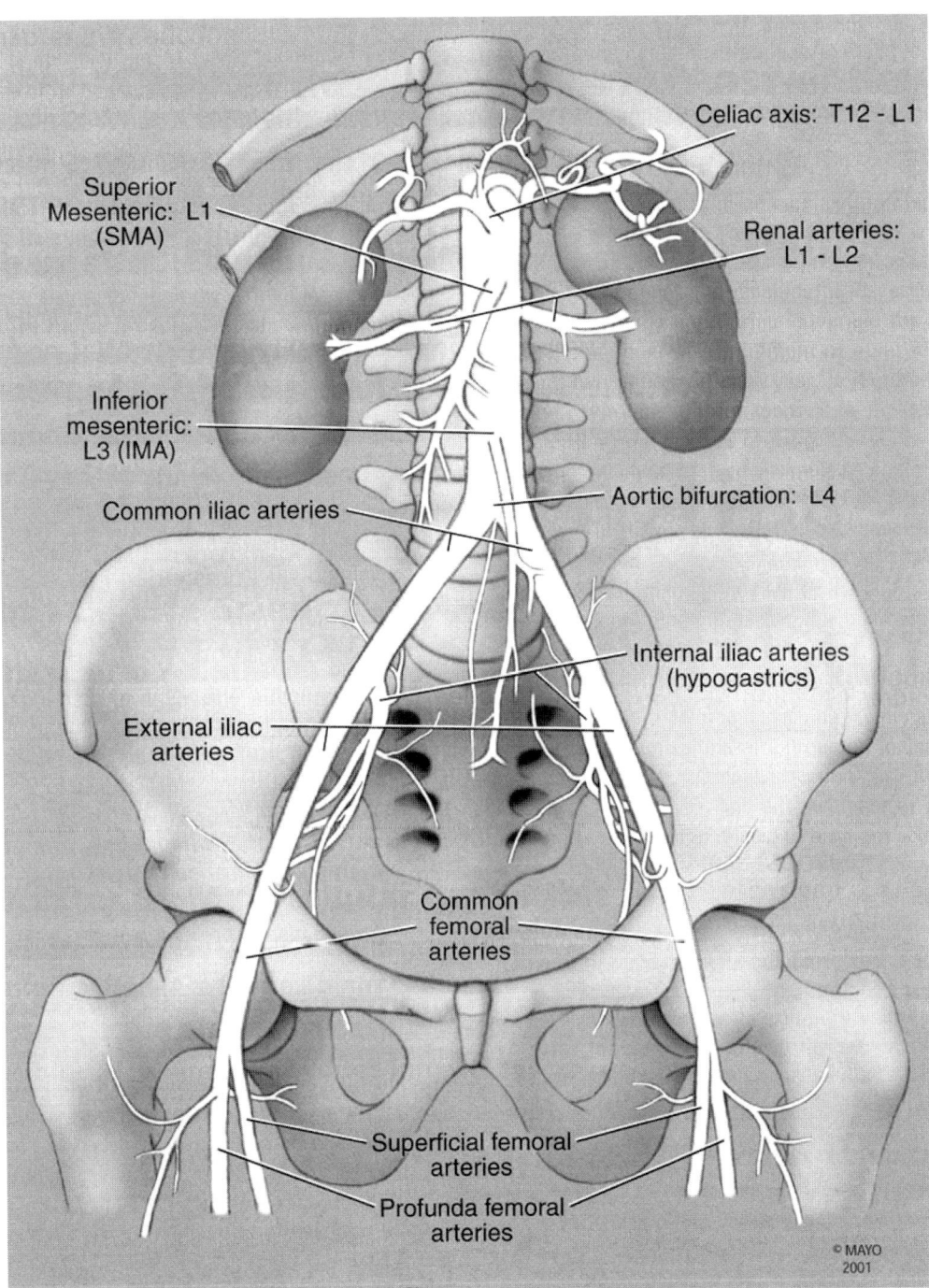

Fig. 56. Abdominal aorta and iliac arteries.

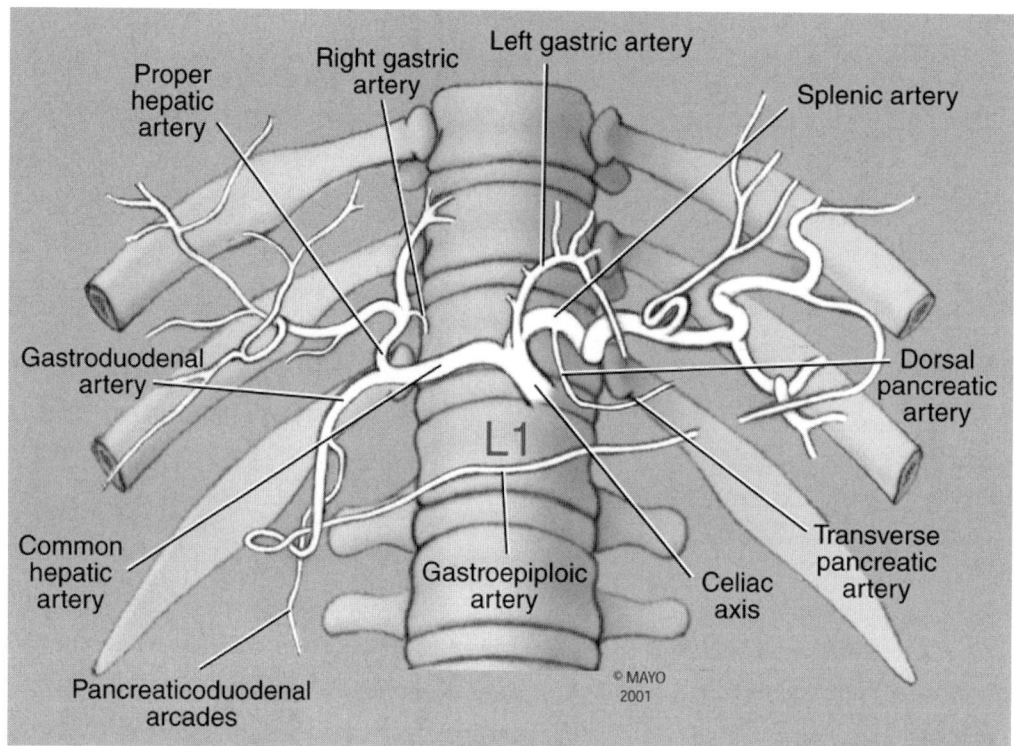

Fig. 57. Celiac axis.

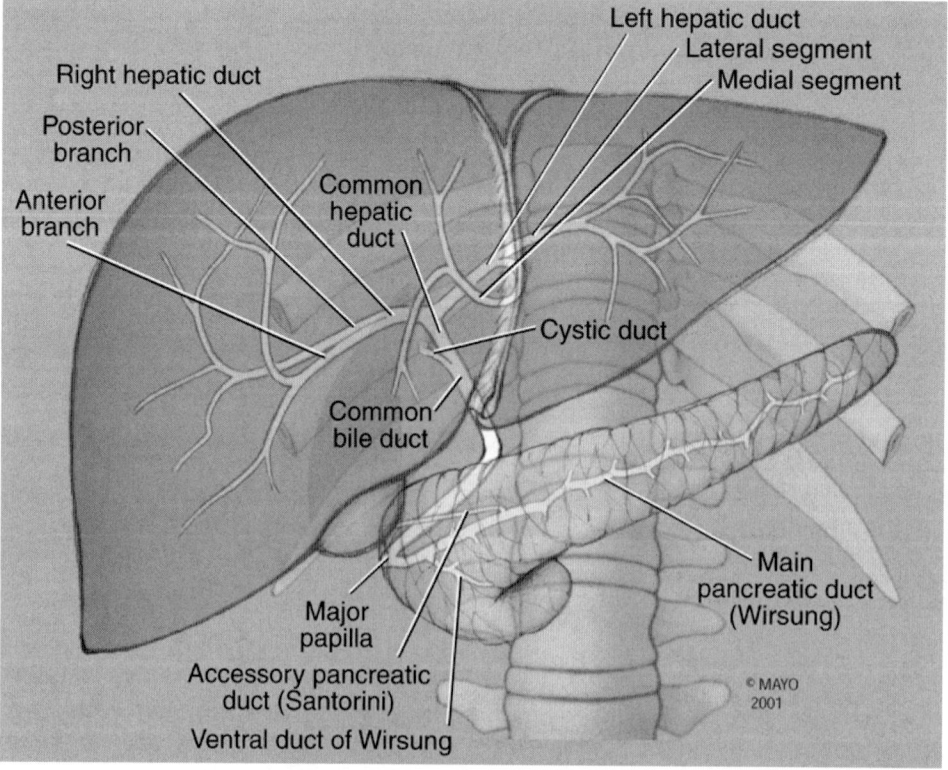

Fig. 58. Biliary and pancreatic ductal system.

5 Neurovascular Angiography

Before the widespread use of cross-sectional imaging, cerebral angiography was one of the most common diagnostic procedures in diagnostic radiology. With the advent of CT and MRI in the 1970s and 1980s, the exquisite anatomic and diagnostic information obtained from these examinations began to confine the role of angiography to its core strength of evaluating vascular abnormalities. The maturing of CT and MRI with the widespread use of MR and CT angiography has further encroached on the use of angiography in a primary diagnostic capacity. Furthermore, the dramatic progress in interventional neuroradiologic materials, techniques, and therapies has changed the role of angiography from primarily diagnostic to primarily pretherapeutic or therapeutic. However, the ability to perform a cerebral angiogram rightly remains a core skill in the diagnostic armamentarium of the radiologist.

1 MATERIALS

As mentioned in other sections of this book, the equipment and materials necessary for procedures will vary widely according to the diagnostic needs, procedural experience, and anatomic demands. This is neither an all-inclusive list nor a list of recommended materials but rather gives examples of basic types of equipment used in cerebral angiography.

Needles

Angiographic puncture needles are generally of two types, single-wall and double-wall. These range in size from 16 to 22 gage and from 5.5 to 10 cm in length, with 18 gage and 5.5 cm the usual size. Single-wall needles were designed with the intent that only the superficial wall of the vessel be punctured. Although they are routinely used for general vascular access,

single-wall needles are particularly helpful when access site hemorrhage is of greater concern. Examples include thrombolysis, a bleeding diathesis, and supranormal anticoagulation. Double-wall needles are styletted with only a small internal channel to allow back-bleeding. These were designed for greater safety in intravascular placement. Both the superficial and deep walls of the artery are designed to be punctured, at which time the stylet is removed and the needle withdrawn until good back-bleeding is noted. This ideally allows for more accurate placement of the needle tip in the center of the lumen and ideally decreases the risk of vessel injury from wire and needle manipulation. Regardless of the design strengths of these needles, one should become proficient with at least one of the two types.

DOUBLE-WALL

Potts, Potts-Cournand, and Modified Potts-Cournand (Fig. 14)

– Variations on the same theme of a beveled needle with a perforated stylet
– Accepts 0.035-inch wires when stylet removed.

Amplatz

– A very utilitarian needle, not just for vascular access
– A three-part beveled needle with occlusive trocar and outer silastic intracath. If the occlusive trocar is removed, the orifice will accept 0.018-inch wires for modified Seldinger technique or a Luer-lock attachment. The outer Silastic intracath can be advanced over the needle into the vessel and can accept 0.035-inch wires and a Luer-lock attachment.

SINGLE-WALL

– An 18-g needle will accept 0.035-inch wires and Luer-lock tip.

MICROPUNCTURE (FIG. 16)

—A wonderful access set with value when hemorrhage is of great concern, as in brachial artery punctures. It is very useful in pediatric patients, as the smaller needle may prevent the vessel spasm that occurs all too frequently in this patient population. The typical set contains a 21-g, 4-cm needle, a 40-cm, 0.018-inch, floppy-tipped wire, and a 4-Fr coaxial 10-cm catheter, which accepts an 0.035-inch wire. This can then be exchanged for a regular sheath.

Wires

Wires used in cerebral angiography are the same as those used for peripheral angiography. However, when catheterizing the cervical vessels, only floppy-tipped or angled-tip wires are typically used.

TEFLON COATED

Bentson (Fig. 2)

– 145-cm length
– A standard wire for vascular access and selective catheterization
– A straight 0.035-inch wire with a 15-cm floppy tip, which leads advancement to prevent dissection.

J-Wire

– 145-cm standard length
– A 180-degree curve at the leading edge of a straight 0.035-inch wire. The blunt curve leads wire advancement to prevent dissection.
– Available in differing diameter curves. A 15-mm turn is typical for common femoral artery access. A tight J-wire with a 3-mm turn is very safe and useful in atherosclerotic vessels

Exchange Length Wires

– Amplatz Stiff, Amplatz Extra Stiff, Amplatz Super Stiff
– 300-cm, 0.038-inch wires in varying degrees of stiffness that are used for catheter exchanges when loss of position in the subselected vessel is feared
– Not designed for primary vascular access or routine wire/catheter manipulation.

HYDROPHILIC COATED

Angled Glidewire (Fig. 3)

– A 145-cm, 0.035-inch hydrophilic-coated wire. It is used for crossing stenoses and selective/subselective catheterizations because of the excellent directional control and slippery hydrophilic coating. Accurate control often requires use of a torque device because of the extremely slippery coating. This wire, as well as any catheter with this type of coating, needs to be preflushed and wiped with saline before each use.

Catheters

There is great variation not only in catheter shape but also in stiffness. It is a general rule in interventional procedures that "softer is better," referring to the tools and materials used. Common sense would seem to indicate that the fewer traumas induced by catheters and wires that are more pliable than others would lead to fewer complications. Alternatively, it can be very difficult to catheterize some vessels without a certain degree of catheter stiffness to transmit the desired movements from fingers to catheter tip. Similarly, catheters and wires should be relatively matched in stiffness for optimal functioning of the pair.

SIMPLE CURVE TYPE

"Pinky" (Fig. 59)

– A 100-cm straight catheter made of polyethylene with a 45-degree angle to the terminal 1 cm. It accepts 0.035-inch wires. Made by Cook, this catheter is a favorite at certain institutions such as the Mayo Clinic and is the softest catheter of the group. It has less than 1:1 torque control, and one must become accustomed to the tactile response of the catheter to maximize its utility, but the catheter's softness gives it a very low complication rate. It is often advanced without a wire into the cervical vessels.

45° Glidecath (Fig. 60)

– A 5-Fr, 100-cm catheter with a similar 45-degree angle to the terminal 1 cm. It accepts 0.035-inch wires. It is made by Terumo but is nearly as soft as the "Pinky" catheter. It has a slippery hydrophilic coating and a 1:1 torque ratio, for excellent control. It is often advanced into the cervical vessels without a wire.

Mayo DAV (Fig. 61)

– 5-Fr, 100-cm catheter with 15-cm bonded soft tip. Accepts 0.035-inch wire.

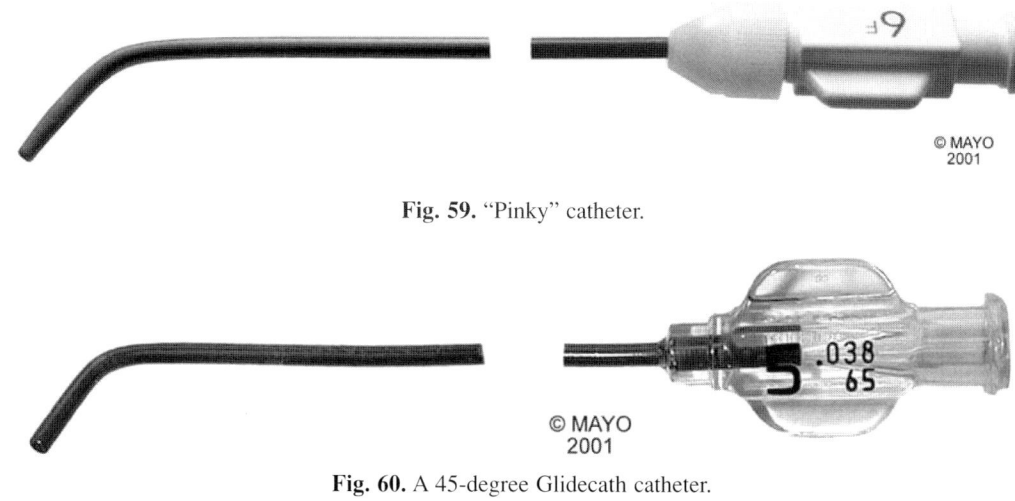

Fig. 59. "Pinky" catheter.

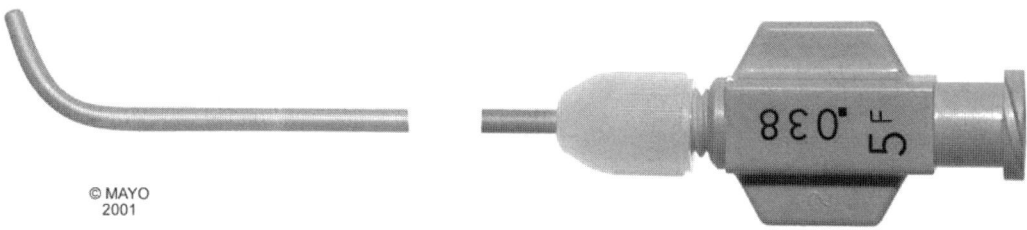

Fig. 60. A 45-degree Glidecath catheter.

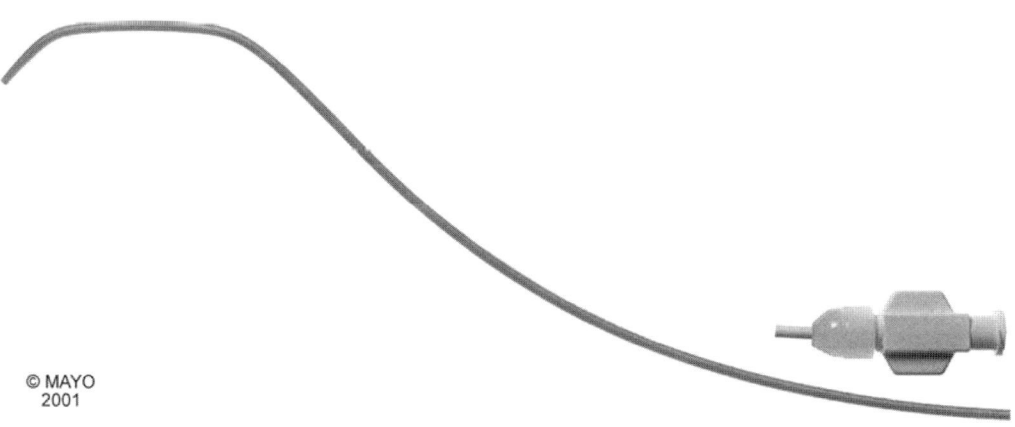

Fig. 61. Mayo DAV catheter.

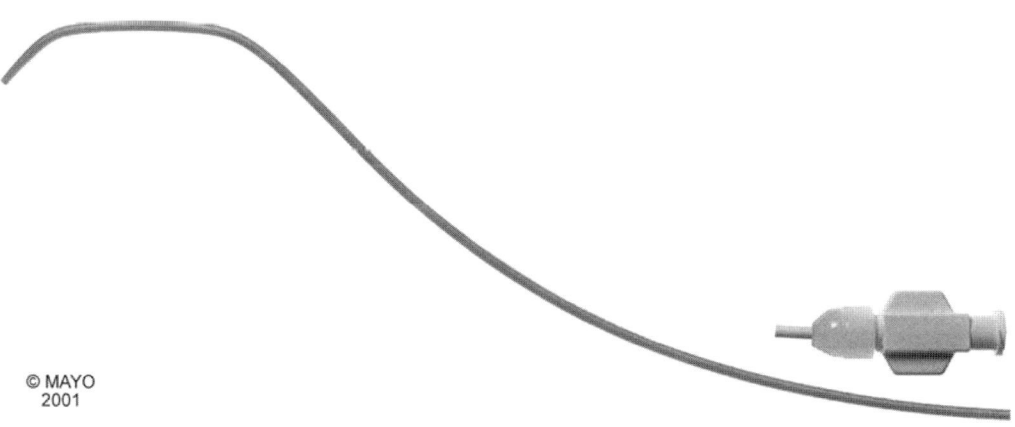

Fig. 62. Headhunter catheter.

DAV-A1

−5-Fr, 100-cm catheter with 3-cm bonded soft tip. Accepts 0.035-inch wire.

Headhunter (Fig. 62)

−5-Fr, 100-cm catheter available with and without a hydrophilic coating. Its shape is reminiscent of cobra-style catheters; this shape is thought to be advantageous in catheterizing the great vessels. It is a stiffer catheter than the simple curve catheters mentioned above. It is usually advanced over a wire. This is thought to be the most common catheter used for neuroangiography. It accepts a 0.035-inch wire.

COMPLEX CURVE

Sidewinder (Simmons, Fig. 29–30)

−5-Fr, 100-cm catheters shaped like a saxophone. These are very useful in tortuous arches with acute angles to the great vessel origins, which often prohibit catheterization, even with the aid of a wire. Its use requires formation of the terminal hairpin curve inside the aorta. Several methods are recognized, including forming the catheter over the aortic bifurcation, in the left subclavian artery origin, in a large aortic lumen, and by reflecting the tip off of the aortic valve. The Simmons 2 type is very useful to start with in a tough case. One nice variant is the Simmons Glidecath, available in the 1,

2, and 3 styles. Wonderful illustrations and discussion can be found in either Dr. Osborne's or Dr. Morris' texts on angiography.

Sheaths

A 5-Fr, 11–13-cm sheath with an inner dilator *(Fig. 21)* is the most common choice for cerebral angiography. Larger sheaths are frequently used for neurointerventional procedures. Longer, 25-cm sheaths are available and can be useful in patients with tortuous iliac vessels, as they reduce the number of friction-producing contact points between the catheter and the tortuous vessel walls, allowing for greater torque control. Many manufacturers make these products.

Closure Devices for Hemostasis

Multiple closure devices are available on the market both as individual units and as combination units with certain catheters. These can be very useful in the outpatient setting by reducing the amount of observation time required before discharge. In addition, several of the devices can be used in the face of full anticoagulation, thereby alleviating prolonged manual compressions. They are of two general types. The first and most widely used is a suture closure device that seals the arteriotomy. The other type is occlusive and seals the arteriotomy by approximating a patch along the needle tract. As these are relatively new, there is much variation and innovation, with new styles and variations entering the market.

2 GENERAL PREPARATION

Room Requirements

Monitoring

Electrocardiogram (ECG), pulse oximetry, and automatic blood pressure monitoring are required at a minimum. At some institutions, the pressure waveforms from both the sheath and catheter tip are monitored via pressure transducers attached to the closed flush system. This allows for real-time evaluation of the local environment at the catheter tip; catheter malposition or malfunction can be detected quickly.

Work Table

A standard setup contains a large bowl partially filled with sterile saline and the initial selection of tools, including sheath, wire, catheter, needle, several syringes, waste fluid receptacle, towels, 4 × 4s, and a sharps box for safe needle and blade isolation. The use of a combination continuous flush and injection tubing system is advised for both the catheter and the sheath. Many commercial models are available. They decrease the likelihood of clot formation on or in the catheter, and they limit exposure to the atmosphere and the possibility of injecting a bubble introduced by the many syringe exchanges needed for the traditional double-flush technique. Additionally, pressure transducers can be placed in the continuous flush circuit.

Personnel

At a minimum, the physician, the technologist, and a nurse should be present. Procedures that are more advanced and/or more complex may require the presence of a anesthesiologist or other additional personnel.

Patient Preparation

Preprocedure Preparation

The patient should be npo after midnight and should have normal lab values if possible. However, many of these procedures are performed emergently, and these desirable conditions cannot always be met. Shaving both groin areas is required to reduce the possibility of infection. A Foley catheter is helpful for extended procedures as it increases patient comfort and consequently decreases motion on the images. Documentation of informed consent and a preprocedure preparation should be on the chart. A basic neurologic examination should be performed, and the pulses (femoral, dorsalis pedis, and posterior tibial) should be palpated on both sides. A review of the patient history and chart is mandatory.

Table Preparation

A sterile Betadine® scrub of both groin areas when the patient is on the table should be performed before sterile draping with a standard angiographic drape.

3 THE PROCEDURE

The Puncture

Retrograde Femoral Artery Puncture

Retrograde common femoral artery catheterization is the most common and is considered the safest type of arterial access for cerebral angiography. Following sterile prep and drape over the groin, the exact site of skin puncture and vessel puncture should be localized. Vessel puncture should be performed at the level of the junction between the middle and inferior thirds of the circular femoral head. The reasoning behind this is that this location reliably allows arterial access below the inguinal ligament. Hematomas from punctures above the inguinal ligament have a greater potential space to expand and can lead to significant blood loss and complications. Furthermore, when arterial access is obtained over the femoral head as described above, there is the solid surface of the femoral head to support the femoral artery during postprocedure compression for hemostasis. If arterial access is obtained below the femoral head, there is only muscle and soft tissue deep to the site as the common femoral artery passes medial to the femur. Postprocedure manual compression, can be less successful in this situation since there is no good support for compression, particularly in larger patients. Five seconds of fluoroscopy can accurately identify the vessel puncture level over the femoral head. Cruder methods of identifying the level of the inguinal ligament manually are not recommended, as they fail to localize the inferior margin of the femoral head.

Once the vessel puncture site is determined fluoroscopically, the skin puncture site can be selected. Usually this requires little consideration, but larger patients may require a longer horizontal traverse such that the needle enters the artery at the desired 45-degree angle. Care should be taken to align the skin and vessel puncture sites along the long axis of the common femoral artery. Needle trajectories skew or oblique to the vessel lead to patient discomfort and physician consternation.

One useful technique in the normal-sized patient is to place the fourth or fifth fingers of your left hand over the fluoroscopically identified vessel puncture site and palpate the course of the artery with the rest of your fingers. The ideal skin puncture site is frequently just below your index finger. At this point, avoid moving your left hand during the rest of the puncture procedure. Maintaining this position will avoid searching again for the pulse and will allow more accurate punctures.

Approximately 5 mL of 1% lidocaine without epinephrine is usually sufficient for local anesthesia. A long, 25-g needle is useful. A 1-cm-diameter wheal should be raised in the skin initially at the skin puncture site. The skin contains the clear majority of pain receptors relative to the deeper tissues, and a commensurate amount of local anesthesia should be used. Avoid injecting lidocaine immediately above or adjacent to the artery, as this can cause spasm (particularly in children).

A small skin incision can now be made in the skin wheal. This need not be made any larger than the sheath to be placed but should be deep enough to be through the dermal fascia into the fat. Care must be taken to avoid an arteriotomy, particularly in thin patients. Tenting the skin before the incision may be required.

At this point all that remains is the needle puncture. Either the single-wall or the double-wall technique may be utilized, as previously described. Once good back-bleeding is obtained from the needle, the guidewire can be advanced into the needle. Meticulous care should be taken to avoid moving the needle when the guidewire is introduced. There should be no resistance to advancing the guidewire into the artery. If resistance is encountered, then stop advancing. Subtle repositioning and realigning is often all that is required. If resistance is still encountered, then look under fluoro. Possibilities include everything from dissection to severe arteriosclerosis to occlusion to an errant guidewire either intra- or extravascular. One trick is to remove the guidewire and attempt to reestablish good back-

bleeding. Alternatively, contrast can be injected into the needle as it is manipulated. Once the guidewire is passed into the abdominal aorta to the level of the diaphragm, the needle can be removed. From this point on, control of the wire or catheter at the puncture site must be maintained, particularly when any manipulation is performed. As the needle is removed, the wire should be wiped with a wet 4 × 4. The preflushed sheath/dilator combination is advanced over the wire into the vessel with a gentle twisting motion until it is at its hub. Remove the dilator and wipe the wire.

High Brachial Artery Puncture

If no common femoral artery access is available, or if there is a more proximal aortic abnormality that precludes safe retrograde catheterization, then a brachial artery puncture can be considered. Use of the left arm is preferred, as the catheter will not cross the right common carotid artery origin in the normal patient. This type of puncture carries a greater risk of postprocedure hematoma formation than common femoral artery puncture. The brachial artery is less well fixed in the subcutaneous tissues than the common femoral artery. Because of its mobility, the artery can be a bit of a challenge to puncture well, and it can similarly be difficult to achieve good postprocedure hemostasis. Additionally, and more importantly, any hematoma formation complicating this type of puncture carries significant risk of compressing the brachial plexus. Even small hematomas can cause significant and permanent disability. More traditional (and proximal) axillary artery punctures bring the puncture site closer to the plexus, and a more distal, high brachial artery puncture is recommended. Any postprocedure abnormalities or complaints should be given the highest priority for evaluation after this type of access, as conservative treatment is not an option, and prompt surgical intervention is the rule.

Performing this puncture is straightforward, but attention to detail in the setup and preparation bring the reward of greater success and fewer complications. Ideally, the left arm should be abducted to approx 90 degrees and flexed to a comfortable position, allowing good exposure. Palpate and document the arm and wrist pulses on both arms for a baseline. As the risk of hematoma carries significant ramifications in this location, the use of a micropuncture set is advisable, as is the use of ultrasound guidance. These measures help ensure a good single-wall puncture. Use of the micropuncture set and particularly the use of ultrasound guidance can help localize this mobile artery well and avoid false or tangential needle passes.

Catheterization and Imaging

As with any interventional procedure, catheterization of the cervical vessels can be disarmingly easy or infuriatingly hard. This concept is artfully reflected in the many catheter shapes used in cerebral angiography. The most basic and common types have been described, but there are others with different and unique shapes as well as advanced materials to deal with almost any situation. Numerous presentations, chapters, and entire books have been devoted to descriptions of catheterization technique.

The basic description of the technique of vessel catheterization for a cerebral angiogram will vary from institution to institution. Some neuroradiologists feel that the very soft catheters can be advanced into the cervical vessels without first advancing a wire. Others feel that no catheter should be advanced into any vessel without first passing a wire into the vessel. I believe all would agree that the stiffer catheters should be used with a wire during vessel catheterization. This description is not all-inclusive and assumes a basic familiarity with angiographic technique, positioning, and experience in setting up one of the combination continuous flush and injection tubing systems. This example features the use of the "Pinky" 45-degree angled straight catheter and assumes that all of the appropriate equipment, medication, and personnel are available.

After appropriate room and patient preparation, the right common femoral artery is accessed via an 18-g Potts needle, a Bentson wire is inserted to the level of the abdominal aorta, and a 5-Fr Sheath is placed. It is now time to flush the catheter with saline and thread it onto the guidewire until a few centimeters of wire are beyond the hub. Watching fluoroscopically, advance the wire catheter combination into the ascending aorta and hold the wire fast before it crosses the valve plane (called "pinning the wire"). Continue to advance the catheter independently over the stationary wire until it too is in the ascending aorta above the valve plane. As the wire gives this very soft catheter more stiffness, use this time to rotate the catheter until the tip points cephalad along the greater curvature of the ascending aorta. Remove the wire without moving the catheter, and aspirate blood from the catheter gently to clear it of any clot or debris.

At this point, connect the catheter hub to the combination continuous flush and injection tubing system while you meticulously observe for any bubbles. Aspirate gently from the power injector port on the continuous flush and injection system to evaluate for the presence of bubbles inadvertently introduced into the system during connection. Be sure to flick the connection hard with your finger to make any hidden bubbles dislodge as blood is aspirated into the tubing. Only when you are convinced there are no bubbles present in the tubing should you inject or flush and fluid through the catheter. When all of the connections are made and no bubbles are seen, make sure the stopcock is open to the continuous flush.

Watching fluoroscopically, gently withdraw the catheter until the tip "pops" into the brachiocephalic trunk. Gently advance the catheter and stop if the catheter begins to meet resistance. If the location of the right common carotid artery (or any other vessel during the procedure) is difficult to find, a short test injection of contrast (2 mL) can help. Once the right common carotid artery is safely catheterized, advance the catheter to the C5-C6 level and pull back until the tip is at C6. After checking intraluminal location with a test injection, any digital subtraction angiography (DSA) run can be performed.

A similar technique can be used to catheterize the left common carotid artery, which, assuming normal great vessel anatomy, will be the next vessel the catheter will "pop" into if gently withdrawn into the aortic arch. To catheterize either vertebral artery, advance into either subclavian artery and use test injections to identify the orifice. Advance the catheter gently a few centimeters into the vessel. This can be tricky, as the vertebral arteries are notoriously quick to spasm after a seemingly atraumatic catheterization. Wise angiographers only advance as far into the vertebral artery as needed and do not stay long. Previous neuroradiologic exams from the same patient can often be helpful in identifing the dominant vertebral artery. Injecting the dominant vertebral artery will often allow reflux down the contralateral side to the level of the contralateral posterior inferior cerebellar artery (PICA) origin. This can exclude an aneurysm at the PICA origin and, unless there is a question concerning the proximal contralateral vertebral artery, can obviate the need to catheterize the other vertebral artery.

If you are unsuccessful in your attempts to catheterize a patent vessel, a wire may be needed. Preflush an angled-tip glidewire, and disconnect the catheter hub from the continuous flush system. Advance the wire, and direct the catheter tip at the vessel orifice. If the wire passes into the vessel with no resistance, advance the wire a few centimeters into the vessel. Manually secure the wire, and advance the catheter gently over the wire. If the catheter does not advance easily because of the anatomy encountered, a gentle "jiggling" advancement can be helpful. Withdraw the wire, and aspirate blood with a syringe to make sure you have good flow. After reconnecting to the continuous flush and injection system, a test injection is a good idea to document intraluminal location. Catheterize the vessels you need to, but no more. Safe cerebral angiography requires catheterizing only those vessels necessary for diagnosis.

Injections

Nonionic contrast is recommended for cerebral angiography. Injection rates for cerebral angiography vary depending on many factors including the size of the vessel, the presence of stenosis, the outflow of the vascular bed, catheter position (tenuous or secure), and the pathology. (A high-flow fistula requires a different injection than an aneurysm.) A general rule is that the injection rate for a vessel is approx its diameter in millimeters. The lingo for describing an injection differs from institution to institution, and good communication with the technologist is paramount. Injections are usually described by both a rate and a total volume of the injection (8 mL volume at 6 mL/s), or by a rate and the length of time the injection lasts (5 mL/s for 2 s). On a practical note, an advisable maneuver is to have the patient wiggle both feet and hands and respond verbally after each injection.

Here are some general examples for injection rates in selected vessels.

Vessel	Volume of contrast (mL)	Rate (mL/s)
Aortic arch	30	10
Carotid bifurcation	5	5
Common carotid artery	9	5
Internal carotid artery	7	4
External carotid artery	6	2
Vertebral artery	8	4

Another injection variable that can be manipulated for better images is the linear rate rise function on the power injector. This controls the rate of acceleration of the injection to its terminal velocity over the first second of injection. A standard rate rise is 0.5 s. This can be decreased to prevent a tenuously positioned catheter from being dislodged and wasting an injection.

Imaging

DSA is clearly the dominant form of image acquisition in cerebral angiography. With recent advances, the resolution of DSA now rivals and surpasses that of existing film screen technology. Biplane DSA is preferred, as the total intraarterial contrast dose is more efficiently used and the radiation dose is decreased. The types of views that are generally used include a standard set of views with as many additional views as are nec-

essary to evaluate the pathology accurately and completely. Classically, for a complete diagnostic angiogram, at least two orthogonal views of the intracranial circulation are required from injections of each carotid artery as well as each vertebral artery. This can often be shortened to three vessels if the dominant vertebral artery is injected and there is contrast reflux down the contralateral vertebral artery sufficient to visualize well the contralateral PICA origin. The standard set of images includes AP and lateral views of the carotid bifurcations, a Towne's view/lateral view biplane combination of the head from injections of both common carotid arteries, and Towne's and lateral views of the posterior fossa (such that both PICA origins are visualized) from one and if necessary both vertebral arteries. Occasionally, similar views of subselective catheterizations of the internal and external carotid arteries are needed.

Filming rates are important variables. Different pathologies will require different filming rates to highlight and reflect their dynamic nature accurately. For routine cerebral angiograms (vasculitis, for example), a filming rate of 2 frames/s for the first 4–5 s followed by 1 fr/s *ad infinitum* is usually sufficient. For aneurysm searches and evaluations, a higher rate is needed. Filming at 4 fr/s for the first 3 s followed by 2 fr/s for 1 s with a terminal filming rate of 1 fr/s *ad infinitum* will usually give adequate detail. Higher flow lesions such as carotid-cavernous fistulas may require rates as high as 7 fr/s for adequate evaluation.

4 POSTPROCEDURE CARE

Hemostasis

The traditional and most common method is hands on. Manual compression of the common femoral artery puncture site has stood the test of time. A recommended method involves aligning the fingers of your left hand along the course of the common femoral artery in a similar manner as you made the puncture. The ring or middle finger is placed over the location of the vessel puncture site, and the sheath passes under your first finger as it enters the skin. As the sheath is smoothly removed, pressure is

applied by the fingertips. Pressure should be nonocclusive, and a pulse should be palpable at all times. The aim is to occlude the arteriotomy and not the vessel. Having one or two fingers above the vessel puncture site will help to decrease the inflow slightly to the region of the arteriotomy. Holding the pressure for 10–20 min is usually sufficient. The patient should have orders written for bed rest and to lie with the procedure side leg straight for at least 4–6 h after the procedure. After hemostasis, the distal pulses should be evaluated and compared with preprocedure documentation, and a repeat neurologic exam should be performed.

5 VASCULAR ANATOMY

See Figures 63–71.

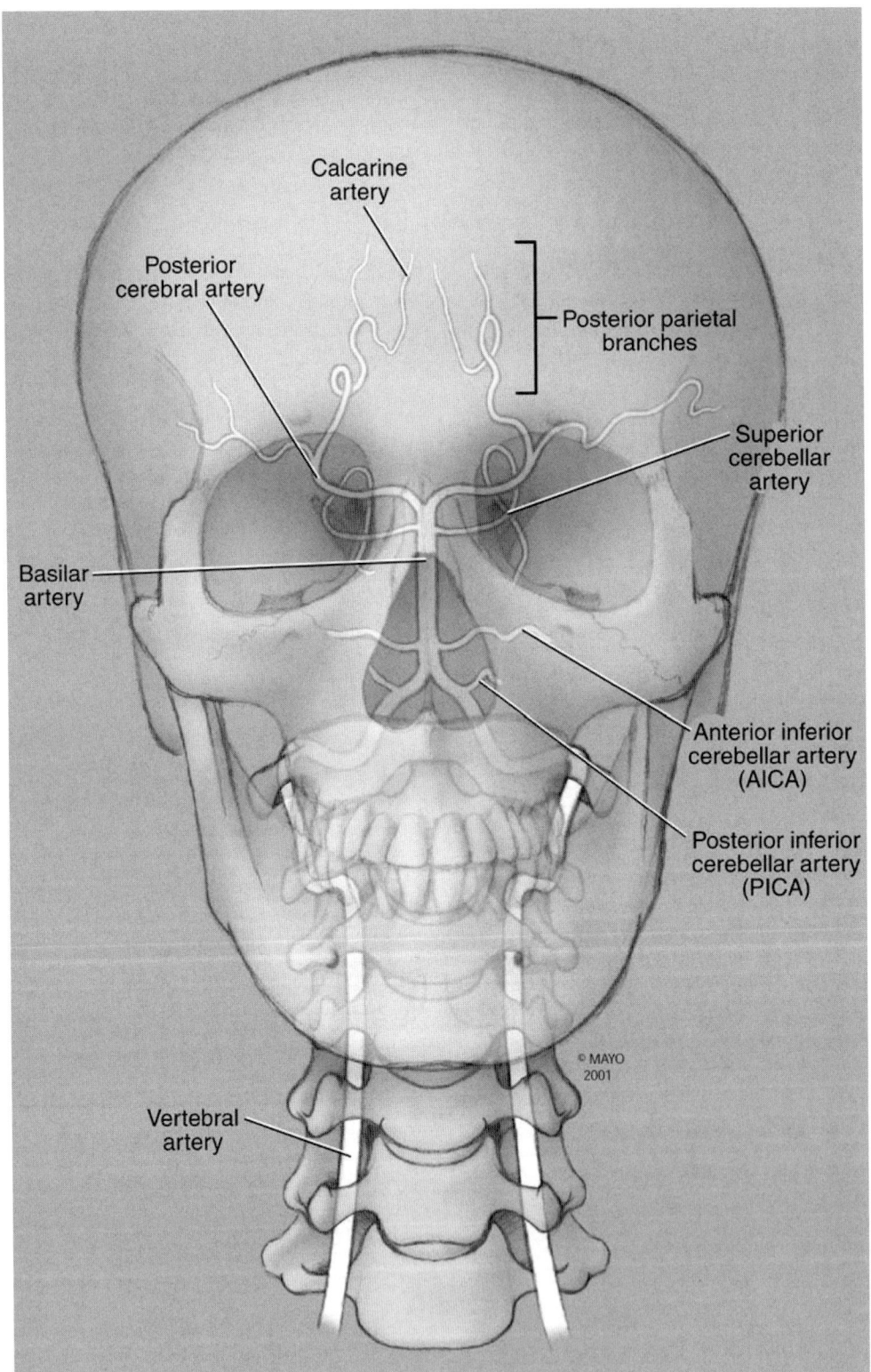

Fig. 63. Vertebral arteries (AP view).

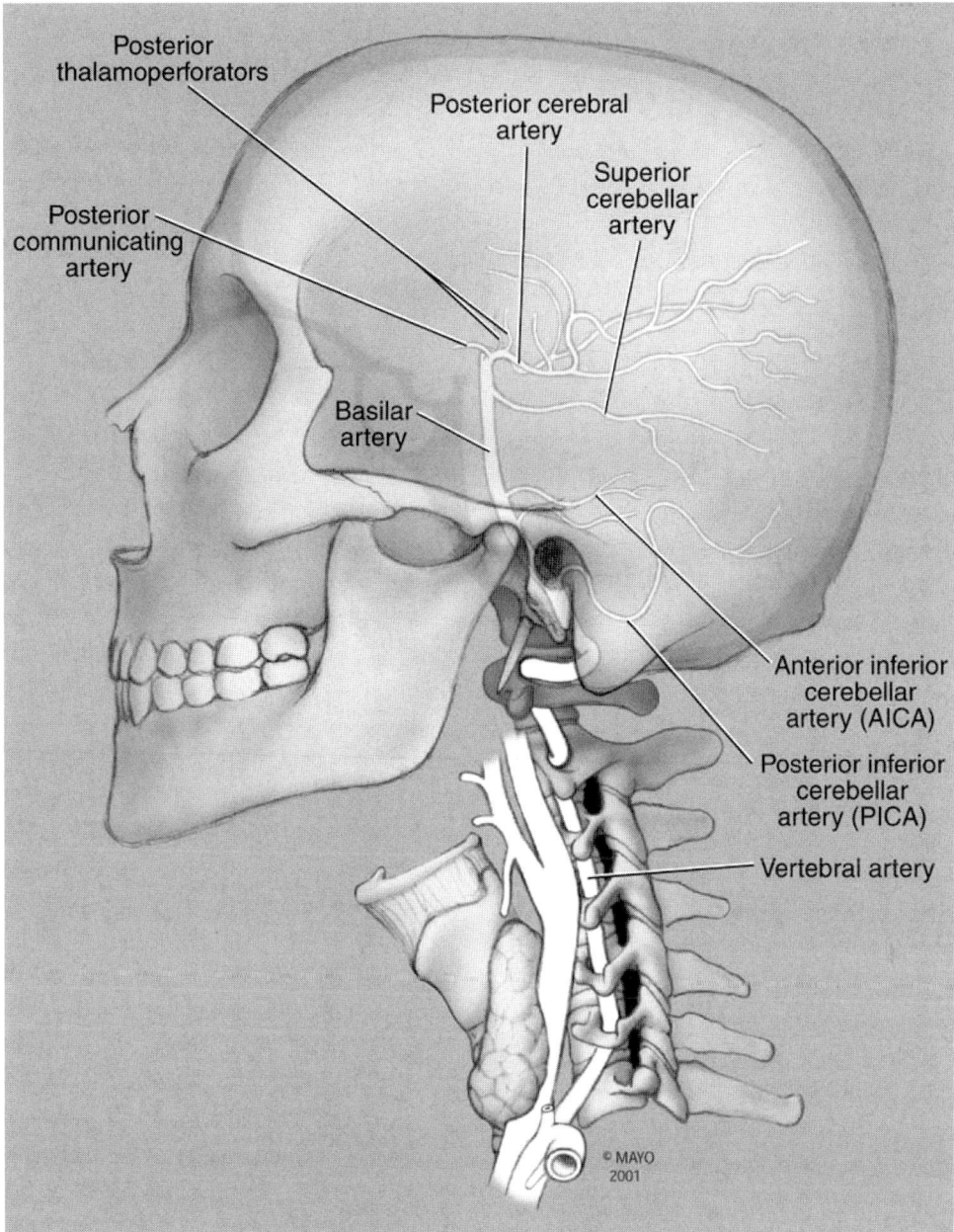

Fig. 64. Vertebral artery (lateral view).

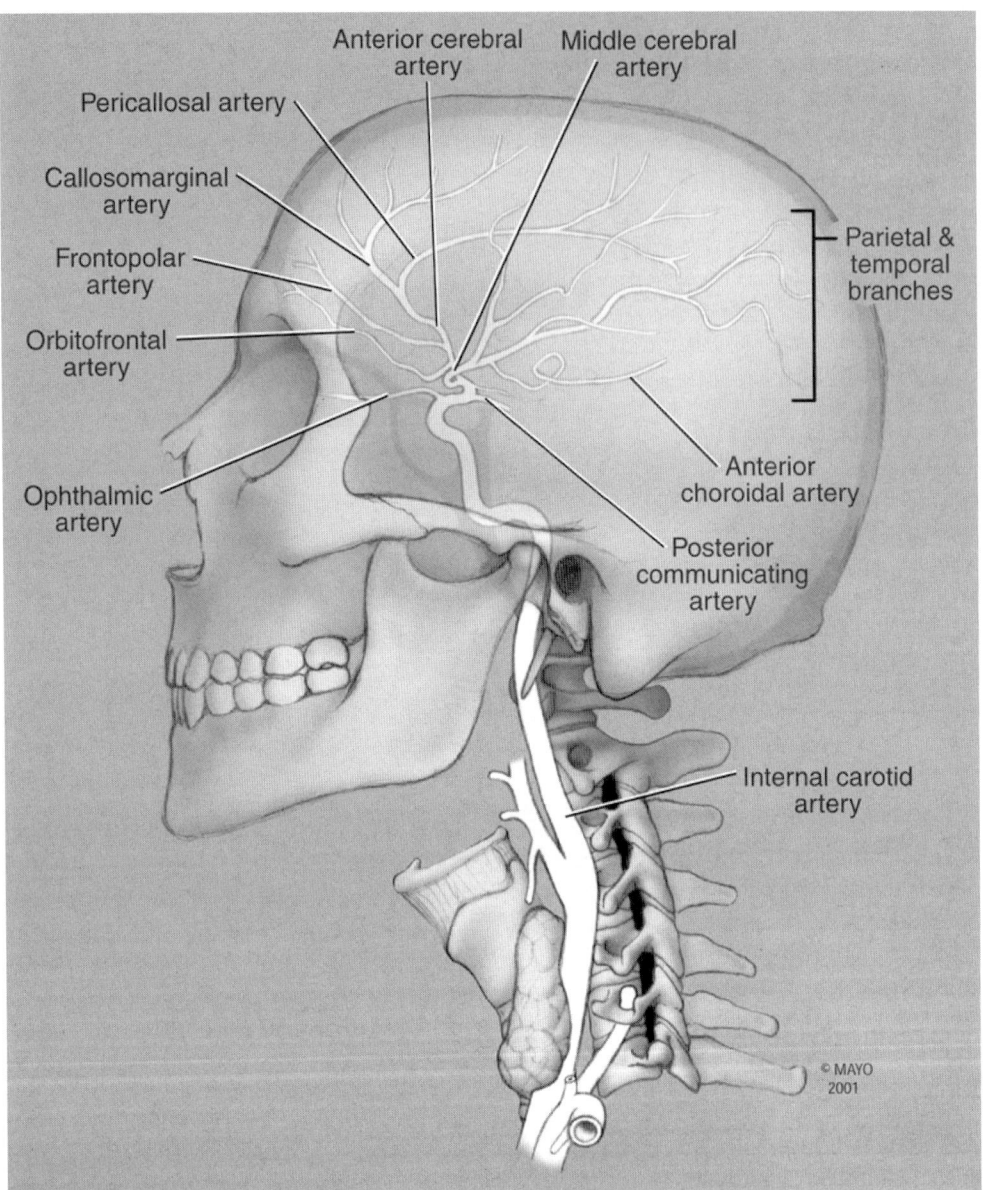

Fig. 65. Internal carotid artery (lateral view).

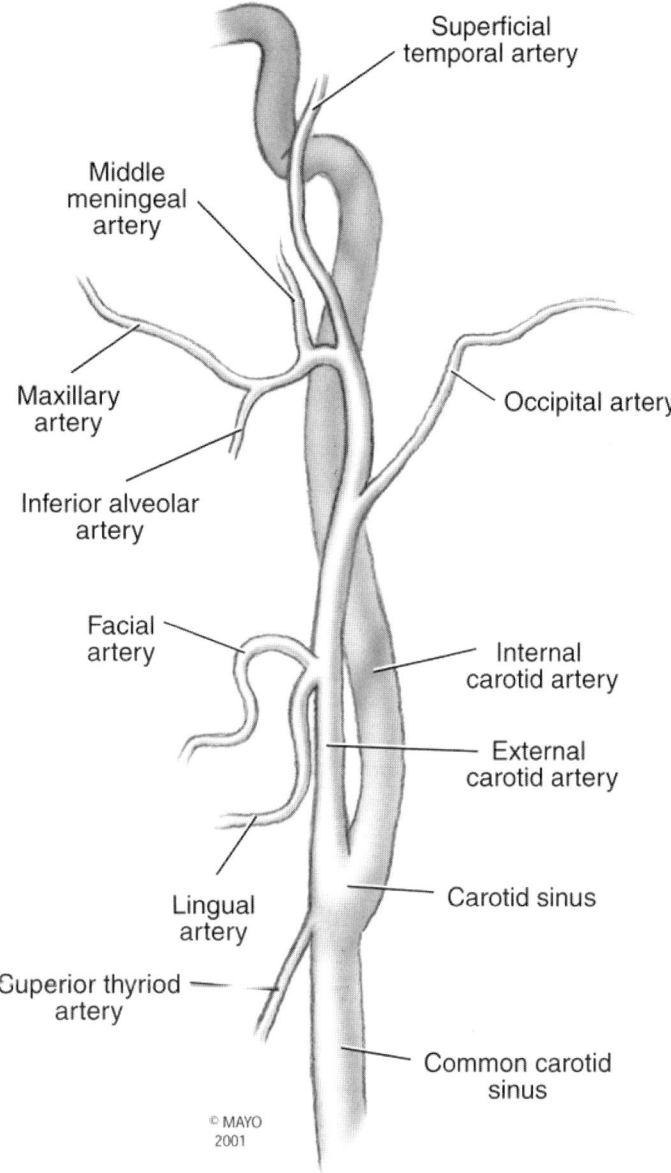

Fig. 66. Carotid arterial circulation at the level of the carotid bifurcation.

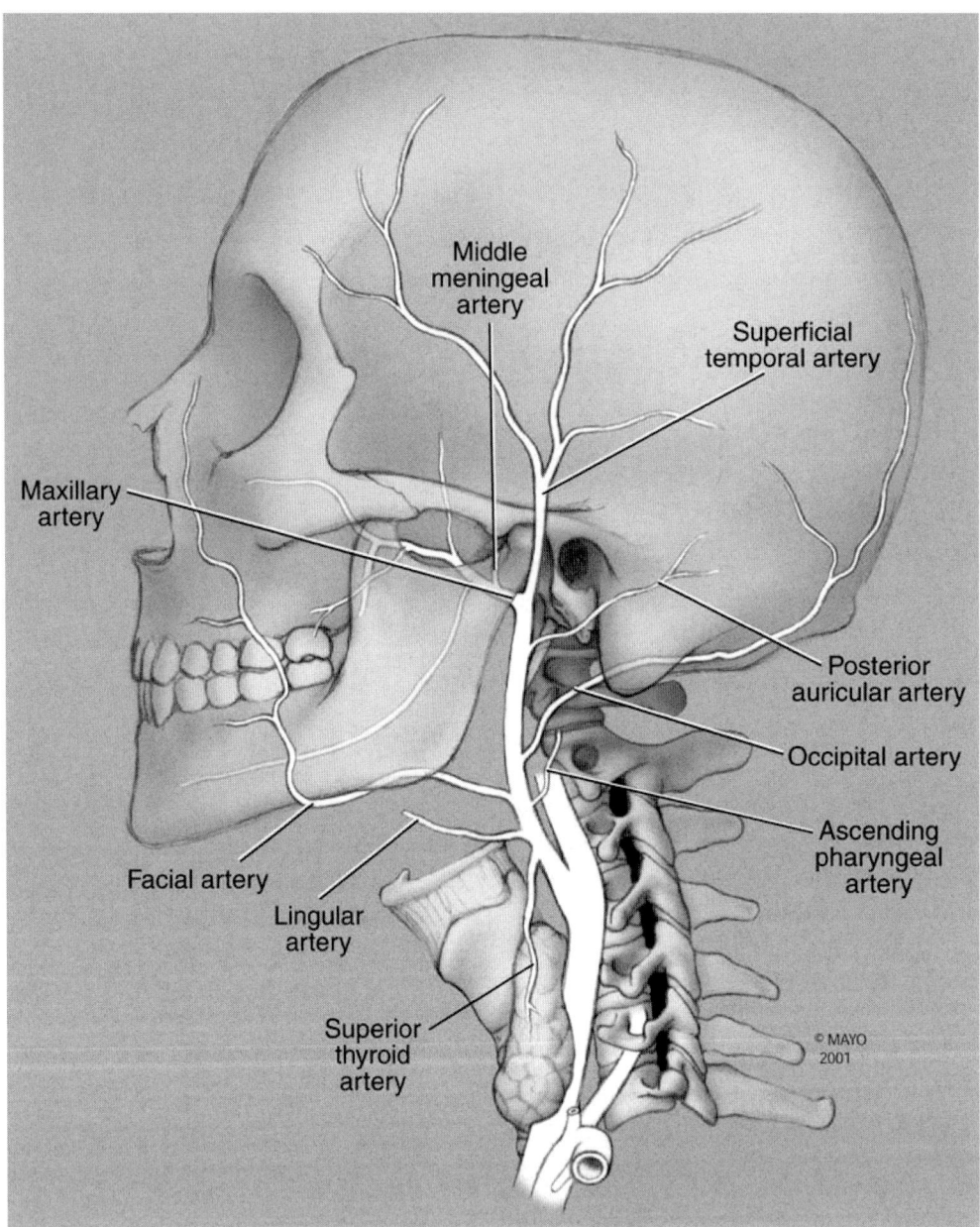

Fig. 67. External carotid artery (lateral view).

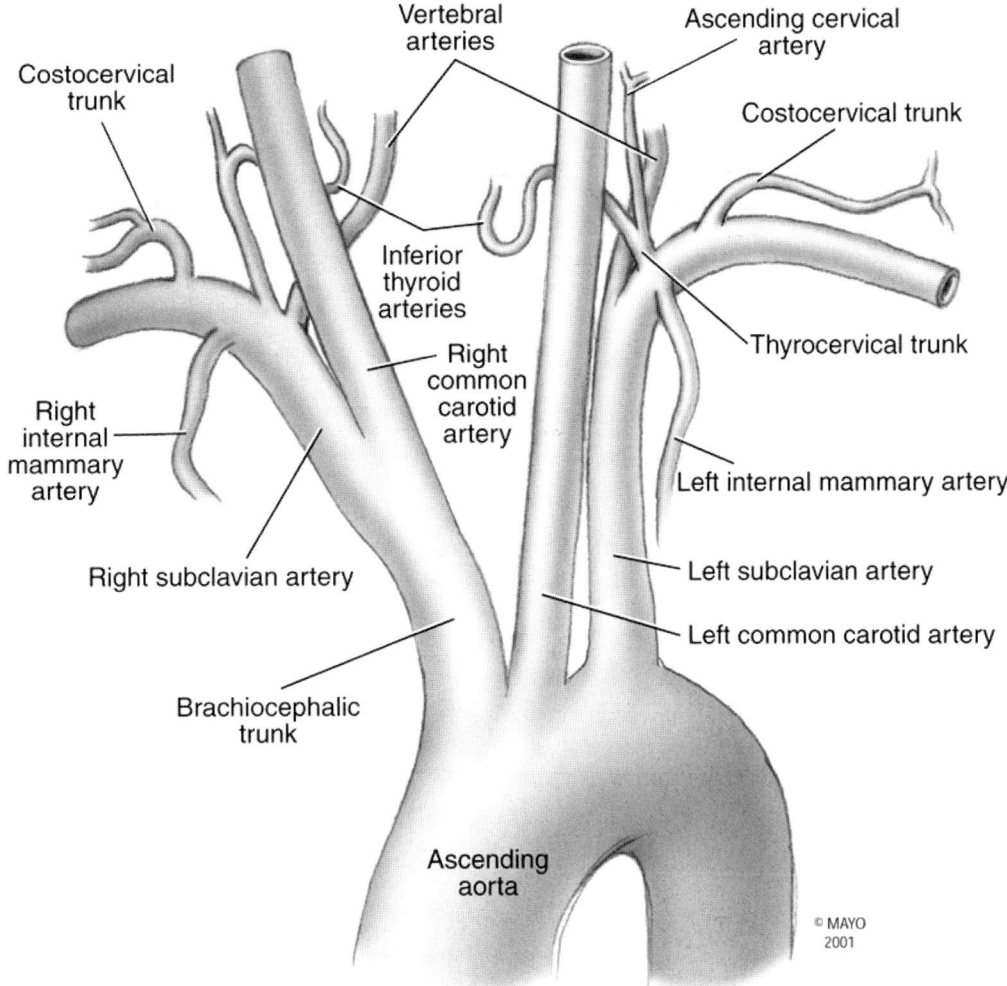

Fig. 68. Aortic arch and great vessels.

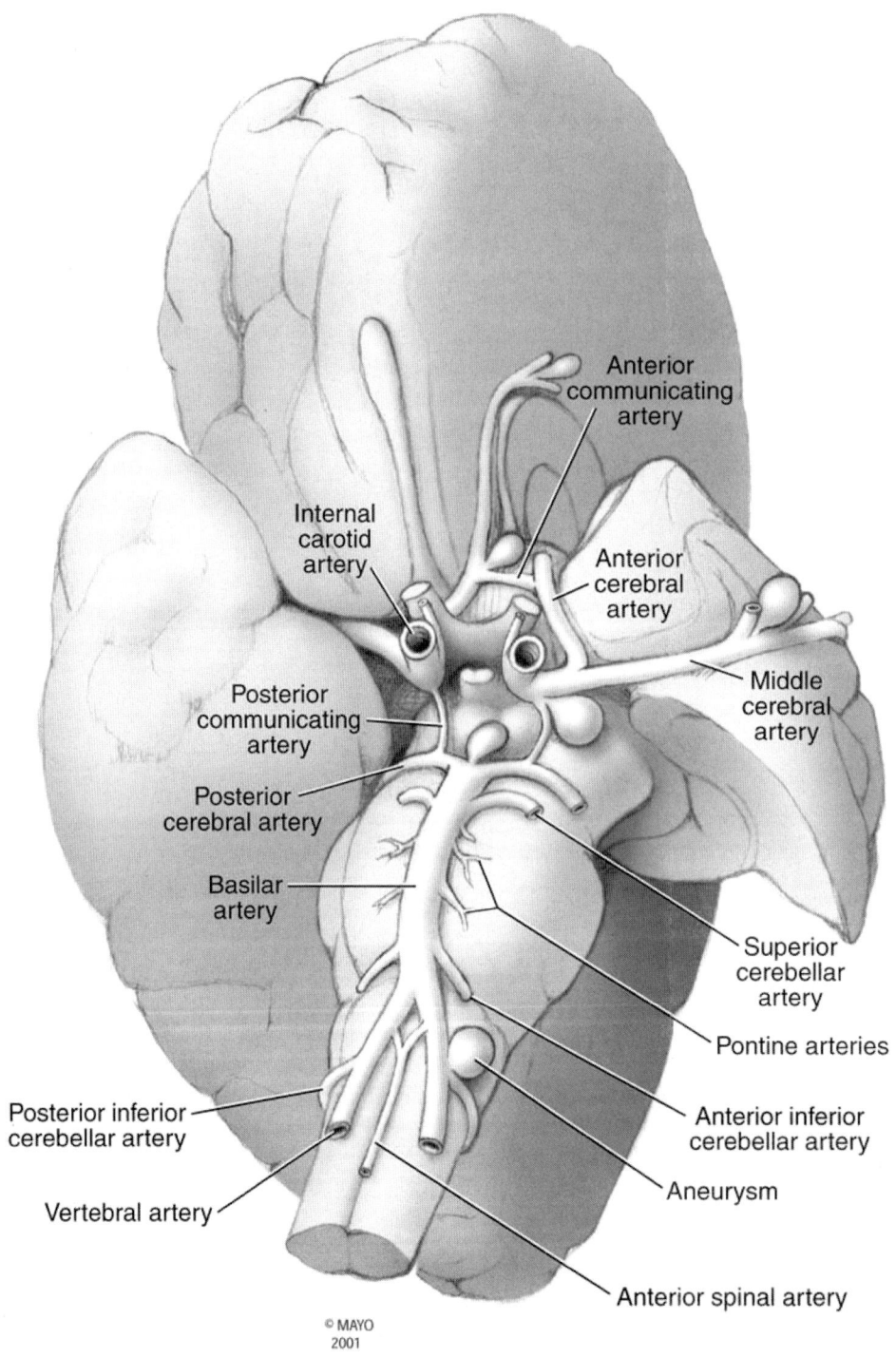

Anterior
communicating
artery

Internal
carotid
artery

Anterior
cerebral
artery

Middle
cerebral
artery

Posterior
communicating
artery

Posterior
cerebral artery

Basilar
artery

Superior
cerebellar
artery

Pontine arteries

Posterior inferior
cerebellar artery

Anterior inferior
cerebellar artery

Vertebral artery

Aneurysm

Anterior spinal artery

© MAYO
2001

Fig. 69. Circle of Willis and multiple aneurysms (demonstrating the most common sites of aneurysm formation).

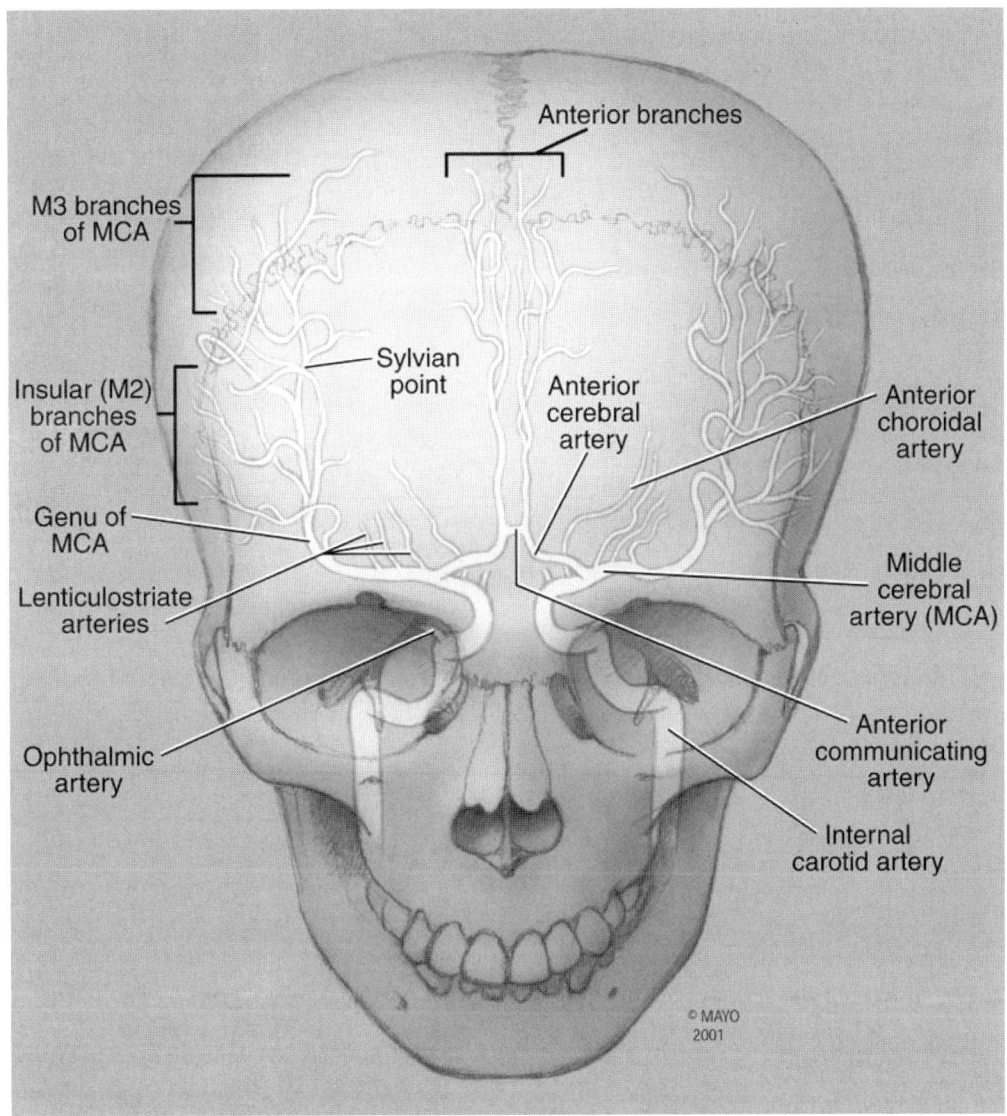

Fig. 70. Internal carotid artery circulation (AP view with 20-degree submentovertex angulation).

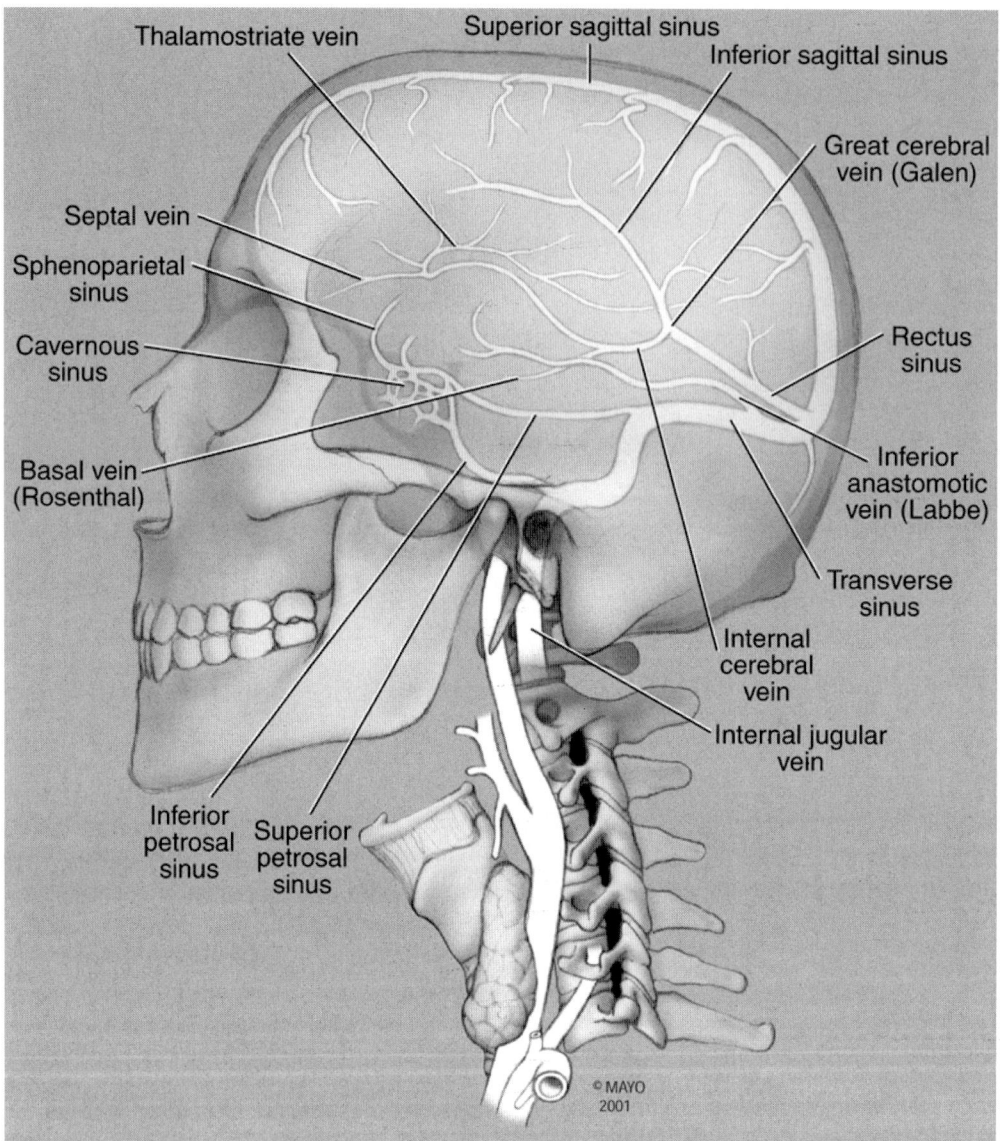

Fig. 71. Intracerebral and dural venous circulation.

6 Film Reporting

PLAIN FILM RADIOGRAPHY

Optimal Reporting Style and Logic

Medical reports not only communicate medical information but are legal documents subject to critical scrutiny. They should be logical, concise, and as precise as possible.

Most Important Findings First

The most efficient report is concise and gives the most important findings first. *"Headlining" the most important findings before lesser information eliminates the need for summary impressions.* Traditional reports have description and discussion, ending with impressions (putting most important information last.)

Report Elements

Reports can include six elements:

1. Normal and normal variants
2. Pathology and anatomy
3. Descriptions: extent, size, shape, location, measurement
4. Certainty: possible (<50%)/probable (>50%)/cannot exclude <5%). *"or"* is the simplest way to express uncertainty:
   a. "Mass right upper lobe due to granuloma" *or* "cancer"
   b. "Cardiomegaly" *and/or* "pericardial effusion"
5. Change: appearing/gone/increasing/decreasing/unchanged
6. Advice for further high-yield study.

Data Reduction

Eliminate needless words by:

1. Concise telegraphic style
2. Using diagnoses instead of descriptions
3. Accentuating the positive and eliminating negative information.

Example

"There is an enormous mass in the right upper lobe" reduces to: "20-cm mass RUL."

Abbreviations, like codes, reduce data but must be universally understood.

Normals, Disease, and Significance

Radiology reports must give useful information for patient care and fall into three main categories:

Normal (no abnormality)
Normal except for non-life-threatening findings
Pathology-anatomy with any changes since last exam.

This is analogous to mammographic coding systems that reduce all findings to just 5 digits:

1 = normal
2 = benign disease (i.e., normal except for)
3 = possible cancer (i.e., possible pathology)
4 = probable cancer (i.e., probable pathology)
5 = cancer (i.e., definite pathology)

Advice

Advice for further study to decrease uncertainty should be high yield and cost efficient.

Communications Theory

Communications theory shows that transferring information from a message source is most efficient when "fewer binary digits per character or per unit of time" are used. The optimized report fits this concept and saves time and money.

Template Reports

Canned reports used for normals and simple pathology generate "noise" and mimic the traditional dictated format. Normals may simply be called "normal" and abnormalities reported succinctly with appropriate adjectives and measurements.

Cumulative Report

Serial X-ray reports on one page (like clinical progress notes) improve quality and efficiency for both the radiologist and clinical staff. Concise style increases the number of studies on one page. Quality assurance requires feedback, and this format is ideal for follow-up studies because it offers ongoing audit of prior information and the potential for continuous quality improvement.

7 Sample Dictations

Frequently, to satisfy some institutional preferences or billing requirements for reporting, a traditional dictation with descriptive findings and an impression is necessary. Some sample dictations that may facilitate the process of reporting normal examinations are given below.

1 GASTROINTESTINAL RADIOLOGY

Swallowing Study and Pharyngo-Esophagogram

Clinical history: Coughing spells while eating. Recent aspiration pneumonia.

Technique: The patient swallowed thin barium, thick barium, and barium paste on a cracker, in the AP and lateral positions.

Findings: Oral and pharyngeal structure and function appear normal. Esophageal structure and function appear normal. There is normal gastric emptying to liquids.

Impression: Normal.

Esophagram

Clinical history: Recent odynophagia.

Findings: Esophageal structure and function are normal.

Impression: Normal.

Upper GI with Small Bowel Follow-Through

Clinical history: Upper abdominal pain with guaiac-positive stools.

Findings: Normal stomach, duodenum, and small bowel. Transit time 45 min from mouth to colon.

Impression: Normal.

Enteroclysis

Clinical history: Chronic, unexplained GI bleeding.

Technique/findings: Signed, informed consent obtained. Following local anesthesia to the nostrils and pharynx, the enteroclysis tube was inserted into the right nostril and advanced under fluoroscopy, until the tip was near the ligament of Treitz. A 25-mL balloon was filled to anchor the tube tip. Then 250 mL of Entero H barium, followed by 1000 mL of methylcellulose, was infused into the small bowel. No masses, areas of narrowing, or adhesions were demonstrated.

Impression: Normal.

Whipple Study

Clinical history: Status post Whipple procedure for cancer of the pancreas.

Technique/findings: T-tube cholangiogram, followed by a limited water-soluble contrast upper GI examination, was performed. The hepatico-jejunostomy is patent, without evidence for extravasation. The pancreatico-jejunostomy does not show evidence of extravasation. The upper GI exam demonstrates a patent duodeno-jejunostomy without evidence for extravasation. There is normal gastric emptying.

Impression: Normal.

T-Tube Cholangiogram

Clinical history: Status post cholecystectomy and repair of bile leak.

Technique/findings: A few milliliters of sterile, water-soluble contrast was injected via gravity into the T-tube, demonstrating normal emptying into the duodenum with no evidence for extravasation. No filling defects are seen.

Impression: Normal.

Barium Enema

Clinical history: Recent 20-pound weight loss with guaiac-positive stools.

Findings: Normal colon, with no evidence of stricture or mass. Contrast refluxed into normal-appearing terminal ileum.

Impression: Normal.

2 GENITOURINARY RADIOLOGY

Intravenous Urogram

Clinical history: Right flank pain with hematuria.

Scout film: Unremarkable, no evidence of radiopaque calculi.

Urogram: After written, informed consent, bolus injection of (fill in the blank) mL of (name of contrast agent) was administered, without adverse effect. Prompt parenchymal enhancement with timely calyceal visualization. Kidneys are normal in size, shape, and position. Normal parenchyma. Normal collecting systems and pelves. Normal ureters and urinary bladder. No significant postvoid residual.

Impression: Normal intravenous urogram.

Voiding Cystourethrogram

Clinical history: Pyelonephritis.

Technique/findings: Bladder was catheterized with a (fill in the blank) French catheter, and the bladder was filled by gravity drip with Cysto-Conray to a capacity of (fill in the blank) mL. The filled urinary bladder showed no abnormality. The patient voided continuously without difficulty, emptying the bladder completely. No vesicoureteral reflux.

Impression: Normal voiding cystourethrogram.

Cystogram

Clinical history: Recent pelvic floor surgery.

Technique/findings: Bladder was catheterized without difficulty with a (fill in the blank) French catheter and the bladder filled by gravity drip with Cysto-Conray to a capacity of (fill in the blank) mL, *or* bladder was filled by gravity drip via the suprapubic tube with Cysto-Conray to a capacity of (fill in the blank) mL. The filled urinary bladder showed no abnormality. No vesicoureteral reflux. Postvoid film showed no significant bladder residual.

Impression: Normal cystogram.

Retrograde Urethrogram

Clinical history: Persistent hematuria with suboptimal IVU.

Technique/findings: Retrograde urethral injection of contrast material outlined and distended the entire urethra revealing no abnormality. Contrast material seen in the bladder.

Impression: Normal retrograde urethrogram.

Retrograde Ureteropyelogram

Clinical history: Status post right pyeloplasty for ureteropelvic junction stenosis.

Technique/findings: Retrograde injection of contrast material through the percutaneous nephrostomy catheter outlined normal right collecting systems, pelvis, and right ureter. Contrast flows freely into the urinary bladder.

Impression: Normal retrograde ureteropyelogram.

3 BODY CT

Spiral Chest CT

Clinical history: Possible mass on recent chest X-ray.

Technique: Spiral CT of the chest was performed after the administration of intravenous contrast, without adverse effect.

Findings: The lung parenchyma is normal. The mediastinal structures are normal. There is no evidence of lymphadenopathy. There is no evidence of pleural or pericardial effusion. The visualized portions of the upper abdomen are unremarkable.

Impression: Normal spiral CT examination of the chest.

Spiral Abdominal CT

Clinical history: Abdominal pain.

Technique: Spiral CT of the abdomen and pelvis was performed after the administration of oral and intravenous contrast, without adverse effect.

Findings: The liver, spleen, and pancreas are normal in appearance. The gallbladder is normal. There is no evidence for biliary ductal dilatation. The kidneys are normal in appearance bilaterally, with no evidence for hydronephrosis. The adrenal glands appear normal. The bladder and bowel is unremarkable. There is no evidence for mass or lymphadenopathy in the abdomen or pelvis. There is no evidence for ascites.

Impression: Normal spiral CT exam of the abdomen or pelvis.

High-Resolution Chest CT

Clinical history: Study is performed to rule out infiltrates.

Technique: High-resolution CT of the chest was performed without contrast.

Findings: The lung parenchyma is normal. There is no evidence for infiltrates. The visualized mediastinal structures are unremarkable. There is no evidence for lymphadenopathy. There is no evidence for pleural or pericardial effusion. The visualized portions of the upper abdomen are unremarkable.

Impression: Normal high-resolution CT exam of the chest.

4 BODY MRI

General Points

1. Refer in a "simple" manner to the pulse sequences as T1-, T2-, or proton density-weighted. Other types of images include gradient echo, cine images, in and out of phase gradient echo images, or inversion recovery images. It is not necessary to discuss features like fat saturation or fast spin echo, unless they are uniquely related to the exam (i.e., fat saturation for a lipoma).
2. All examinations should specify the contrast type and amount and route (iv)
3. If glucagon or L-hyoscyamine (Levsin®) was administered, state this.
4. Specify the type of coil that was used: body, torso, pelvis, extremity, flexible coil, shoulder, head, and so on.

Knee MR

Clinical history: Medial knee pain.

Technique: Axial gradient echo, sagittal proton density, sagittal T2- and coronal T2-weighted images. Knee coil.

Findings: The medial and lateral menisci are normal. The anterior and posterior cruciate ligaments are normal. The collateral ligaments are normal. There is no evidence of bone marrow abnormality. The cartilage surfaces are normal. No joint effusion is present.

Impression: Normal.

Shoulder MR

Clinical history: Rule out rotator cuff tear.

Technique: Axial gradient echo, coronal oblique proton density, coronal oblique T2- and sagittal oblique T2-weighted images. Shoulder coil.

Findings: The supraspinatous tendon and remainder of the rotator cuff is normal. The acromioclavicular joint is normal. The acromion is flat in shape. The glenoid labrum is normal. The humeral head is normal in shape, and there is no bone marrow abnormality or joint effusion.

Impression: Normal.

Abdomen MR

Clinical history: Colon cancer.

Technique: Axial T1, T2, and gradient echo images. Gadolinium (15 mL) administered iv followed by dynamic gradient echo images.

Findings: The liver is normal, with no evidence of mass. The spleen, pancreas, and adrenal glands are normal. The visualized portions of the kidneys are normal. There is no retroperitoneal lymphadenopathy.

Impression: Normal.

5 ULTRASOUND

Abdominal Ultrasound

Clinical history: Right upper quadrant pain.

Findings: The liver is normal in size and echotexture. There are no focal lesions present. The gallbladder is normal, without evidence of wall thickening, calculi, or focal tenderness. Normal common duct measuring _____ mm. No intrahepatic biliary ductal dilation. The pancreas is seen (head, body, and tail) and appears normal. The right kidney measures _____ cm, and the left kidney measures _____ cm in length. No hydronephrosis, calculi, or masses are present. Normal spleen. No ascites.

Impression: Normal abdominal ultrasound.

Right Upper Quadrant Ultrasound

Essentially the same examination, except the spleen and the left kidney are not included.

Renal and Bladder Ultrasound

Clinical history: Rising creatinine.

Findings: The right kidney measures _____ cm, and the left kidney measures _____ cm in length. Neither kidney shows evidence of hydronephrosis, calculi, or mass. The bladder is unremarkable in appearance. The postvoid residual was measured to be _____ mL.

Impression:

1. Normal bilateral renal ultrasound.
2. Normal bladder ultrasound.

Pelvic Ultrasound

Clinical history: Vaginal bleeding, right adnexal fullness and pain.

Findings: Ultrasound examination of the pelvis was performed using transabdominal and endovaginal technique. The uterus measures _____ cm in length, _____ cm in AP, and _____ cm in transverse dimension. The size and echo texture of the uterus are normal. The endometrial thickness measures _____ mm. Both ovaries were visualized and appear normal in size and echotexture. The right ovary measures _____ × _____ × _____ cm, and the left ovary measures _____ × _____ × _____ cm. No adnexal masses or free cul-de-sac fluid was present.

Impression: Normal pelvic ultrasound.

Lower Extremity Doppler Ultrasound

Clinical history: Acute bilateral leg swelling and tenderness.

Findings: There is normal flow, compressibility, and augmentation of the common femoral vein, superficial femoral vein, and popliteal vein bilaterally.

Impression: No evidence of deep venous thrombosis in either lower extremity above the knee.

Ultrasound-Guided Biopsy/Drainage Procedure

Clinical history: Rising liver function tests (LFTs), multiple liver masses on recent abdominal ultrasound.

Procedure: Ultrasound-guided biopsy of liver mass.

Prebiopsy diagnosis: Liver masses.

Postbiopsy diagnosis: Same.

Physicians: (Give the names of the resident and the attending).

Medication: 1 mg midazolam; 50 µg Fentanyl® iv.

Complications: None.

Description of procedure: After informing the patient of the risks, benefits, and alternatives, informed consent was obtained. The liver was evaluated with ultrasound. Multiple lesions were seen in both lobes of the liver. A _____ cm lesion in the (state location of lesion) was selected for biopsy. The skin was prepped and draped in the usual sterile fashion and then anesthetized with 2% lidocaine solution. Subsequently a _____ gage (fill in the needle type) needle was advanced into the lesion under ultrasound guidance using a needle guide, and a sample was obtained using the _____ (state type of technique) technique. The on-site pathologist deemed the sample adequate. The patient was observed for _____ h in the ultrasound department following the procedure. The patient was subsequently discharged with the usual instructions.

Impression: Successful and uneventful biopsy of a (state location of lesion) lesion as described above.

Scrotal and Testicular Ultrasound

Clinical history: Left testicular pain.

Findings: Both testicles are normal. The right testicle measures _____ cm, and the left testicle measures _____ cm. Both epididymetes are also normal.

Impression: Normal scrotal and testicular ultrasound.

Thyroid Ultrasound

Clinical history: Palpable thyroid nodule.

Findings: Both lobes of the thyroid are normal, with homogenous echotexture. The right lobe measures _____ cm in length, _____ in AP, and _____ cm in transverse dimension. The left lobe measures _____ cm in length, _____ in AP, and _____ cm in transverse dimension.

Impression: Normal thyroid ultrasound; no evidence of thyroid nodule.

Liver Duplex Ultrasound

Clinical history: Hepatitis.

Findings: The liver is normal in echotexture. Normal hepatopedal flow is demonstrated in the main, right, and left portal veins. Normal flow is also demonstrated in the hepatic artery, in all three hepatic veins, and in the inferior vena cava. The gallbladder is normal. The common duct measures _____ mm, which is normal. There is no evidence of intrahepatic biliary ductal dilation. The right kidney measures _____ cm in length, without evidence of hydronephrosis.

Impression: Normal liver duplex ultrasound.

Carotid Duplex Ultrasound

Clinical history: Recent transient ischemic attack.

Findings: There is no evidence for hemodynamically significant stenosis in either internal carotid artery. No significant atherosclerotic plaques are seen. Antegrade flow is demonstrated in both external carotid and vertebral arteries.

Impression: Normal carotid duplex ultrasound.

6 NEURORADIOLOGY

Noncontrast Head CT

Clinical history: Acute-onset left-sided weakness and slurred speech.

Technique: Standard, noncontrast head CT.

Findings: The ventricles and sulci are normal in size, shape, and position. There are no abnormal intra- or extraaxial fluid collections. The brain parenchyma is normal in attenuation, with no evidence of masses, hematoma, or shift of the midline structures. The calvarium is normal in appearance. The visualized paranasal sinuses and mastoid air cells are clear.

Impression: Normal noncontrast head CT.

Head MRI

Clinical history: Acute-onset left-sided weakness and slurred speech.

Technique: The following imaging sequences were obtained: sagittal T1-weighted images, axial T2-weighted images, and 3D time-of-flight magnetic resonance angiography (MRA) through the circle of Willis.

Findings: The ventricles and sulci are normal in size, shape, and position. There are no abnormal intra- or extraaxial fluid collections. The brain parenchyma is normal in signal intensity, with no evidence of masses, hematoma, or shift of the midline structures. There are normal flow voids in the basilar and carotid arteries. The visualized paranasal sinuses and mastoid air cells are clear. 3D time-of-flight MRA through the circle of Willis demonstrates no evidence for narrowing or aneurysms. The source images also demonstrate no abnormality.

Impression: Normal head MRI.

Contrast-Enhanced Head CT and MRI

Please add the following sentence to the findings. "No abnormal areas of enhancement are demonstrated."

Neck CT

Clinical history: Persistent hoarseness.

Technique: CT images in the axial plane were obtained from the level of the frontal sinuses inferiorly to the thoracic inlet following the uneventful administration of intravenous contrast. (Note whether thin-section images were obtained through an area of specific interest.)

Findings: The spaces of the neck are normal in appearance. There are no enlarged lymph nodes or nodes with low-density centers. There are no abnormal areas of enhancement demonstrated.

Impression: Normal contrast-enhanced neck CT.

CT of the Paranasal Sinuses

Clinical history: Chronic frontal headache.

Technique: CT images in the coronal plane from anterior to the frontal sinuses to posteriorly through the sphenoid sinus.

Findings: The paranasal sinuses are clear. There is no evidence for air-fluid levels or bony erosions. The osteomeatal unit complexes are patent bilaterally.

Impression: Normal CT of the paranasal sinuses.

MRI of the Lumbosacral Spine

Clinical history: Bilateral radiculopathy.

Technique: Sagittal T1- and T2-weighted images were performed from the T12 level inferiorly to the S2 level. Axial T1- and T2-weighted images were performed from the L3 level through the S1 level.

Findings: The alignment of the lumbosacral spine is anatomic. There is no evidence of disc herniation. There is a normal disc hydration signal demonstrated. The conus medullaris is normal in signal intensity. Axial images at the L2-L3 level: the spinal canal and neural foramen are adequately patent. Axial images at the L3-L4 level: the spinal canal and neural foramen are adequately patent. Axial images at the L4-L5 level: the spinal canal and neural foramen are adequately patent. Axial images at the L5-S1 level: the spinal canal and neural foramen are adequately patent.

Impression: Normal lumbosacral spine MRI.

Example of spinal pathology: At the L4-L5 level, there is a posterior disc protrusion. This abuts the right traversing L5 nerve root. The nerve roots exit normally, without evidence for impingement bilaterally. At the L5-S1 level, there are ligamentum flavum and facet hypertrophic changes. This combines with a central disc bulge to cause moderate spinal canal stenosis. The exiting nerve roots are impinged on in the region of the subarticular recesses bilaterally.

MRI of the Cervical Spine

Clinical history: Neck pain.

Technique: The following imaging sequences were performed: sagittal T1- and T2-weighted images from the foramen magnum to the T2 level. Axial T2-weighted images from the C2 level inferiorly through the T1 level.

Findings: The cervical spine is anatomic in alignment. There is no evidence of posterior disc protrusions. The spinal canal is adequately patient. No cord signal abnormalities are demonstrated.

Axial images at the C2-C3 level: the spinal canal and neural foramen are adequately patent.

Axial images at the C3-C4 level: the spinal canal and the neural foramen are adequately patent.

Axial images at the C4-C5 level: the spinal canal and the neural foramen are adequately patent.

Axial images at the C5-C6 level: the spinal canal and the neural foramen are adequately patent.

Axial images at the C6-C7 level: the spinal canal and the neural foramen are adequately patent.

Axial images at the C7-T1 level: the spinal canal and the neural foramen are adequately patent.

Impression: Normal cervical spine MRI.

Plain Film Myelogram

Clinical history: Bilateral radiculopathy.

Technique: After explanation of the risks and benefits of the procedure, informed consent was obtained. Using fluoroscopic guidance, the L2-L3 level was localized. With a 22-g needle, the thecal sac was entered without difficulty (with the stylet in place). The stylet was removed and ___ mL of (name of the contrast agent) was introduced without difficulty. Plain film myelography was then performed.

Findings: The thecal sac is normal in appearance. There is no evidence of disc herniation or spinal canal stenosis. The traversing and exiting nerve roots demonstrate no evidence of impingement. The region of the conus medularis is normal in appearance.

Impression: Normal plain film myelogram of the lumbar spine.

Carotid Angiogram

Clinical history: Recent transient ischemic attacks.

Findings: Common carotid injection reveals no abnormalities of the cervical portions of the carotid artery, including the carotid bifurcation. The bony portions of the internal carotid artery are unremarkable. The supraclinoid internal carotid artery and its branches are also unremarkable. The proximal middle cerebral artery, including its lenticulostriate branches, are within normal limits. The Sylvian vessels, including the image of the Sylvian triangle in the frontal and lateral projections, are normal. There is normal character and distribution of the peripheral branches of the middle cerebral artery. The horizontal segment of the anterior cerebral artery is not elevated. The pericallosal artery is midline and has a normal sweep about the corpus callosum. The peripheral branches of the anterior cerebral artery are normal in character, number, and distribution. During the intermediate phase, no abnormal parenchyma stain is seen, nor are there any early draining veins. The internal cerebral vein is midline, and the subependymal veins outline normal ventricles. The convexity veins are normal in number and distribution and reach the inner table of the skull.

Impression: Normal carotid angiogram.

Vertebral Angiogram

Clinical history: Recent transient ischemic attacks.

Findings: Vertebral angiogram does/does not result in reflux down the opposite vertebral artery. There is good opacification of the posterior circulation. The vertebral and basilar arteries are patent and in their usual positions. PICA is normal, including its choroid point, tonsillar branches, and inferior vermian artery, which is midline. AICA is normal on the frontal view. The superior cerebellar arteries are normal, including their midline superior vermian branches. Posterior cerebral arteries do/do not fill from this injection and have a normal number and distribution of peripheral branches.

The thalamoperforate, thalamogeniculate, and posterior choroidal vessels are unremarkable. During the intermediate phase, no abnormal parenchyma stain is seen, nor are there any early draining veins. The anterior pontomesencephalic vein outlines a normal anterior portion of the brainstem, and the superior vermian vein complex, including the precentral cerebellar vein, is likewise normal. The inferior vermian vein is midline. The petrosal veins are normally filled.

Impression: Normal vertebral angiogram.

7 MAMMOGRAPHY

General Points

The mammographic reporting system should follow the American College of Radiology's Breast Image Reporting and Data System (BIRADS®). This reporting system is a collaborative effort between various organizations and is designed to standardize mammographic reporting, to reduce confusion in breast image interpretation, and to facilitate outcome monitoring.

The report should adhere to the following structure:

1. A statement should be made indicating that the mammogram has been compared with previous mammograms (if this has been done) and giving the dates of prior study.

2. A statement regarding the overall composition of the breast:
   a. The breast is almost entirely fat.
   b. There are scattered fibroglandular densities.
   c. The breast tissue is heterogeneously dense. This may lower the sensitivity of mammography.
   d. The breast tissue is extremely dense, which could obscure a lesion on mammography.

3. A clear description of any significant finding should be made. The clinical location of the abnormality should also be stated. This may be in terms of quadrants (i.e., upper outer quadrant of the right breast) or in terms of positions on the clock face (i.e., the 10 o'clock position of the right breast). The abnormality should also be described in relation to its appearance on a previous examination (if a comparison study is available and the lesion was present).

4. An overall summary or impression should be rendered. This impression should fully categorize the abnormalities, and an indeterminate reading should only be given when additional imaging is recommended.
   a. If the reading is indeterminate, a recommendation for additional imaging should be provided.

5. One of the following assignment categories should be added to the report.
   a. *Category 0: Need additional imaging evaluation.* This should be reserved for an examination that needs additional imaging evaluation. This is nearly always used with screening examinations and is rarely be used after a complete imaging workup. A recommendation for additional imaging should be made.
   b. *Category 1: Negative.* Completely normal breasts with nothing worthy of comment.
   c. *Category 2: Benign finding.* The mammogram is negative for suspicious findings but may have certain benign findings (i.e., lipoma, fibroadenoma, intramammary lymph nodes, implants, and so on) that the interpreter feels necessary to describe.
   d. *Category 3: Probably benign finding; short-interval follow-up suggested.* An abnormality placed in this category should have a high likelihood of being benign, but the radiologist may choose to use this intermediate category to establish a lesion's stability. A 6-month interval is usually the recommended time period for a short-term follow-up, but this may be altered according to the opinion of the radiologist.
   e. *Category 4: Suspicious abnormality; biopsy should be considered.* Lesions that don't have the classic characteristics of breast cancer but that are nevertheless suspicious for malignancy should be placed in this category. If possible, the approximate probability of malignancy should be cited to assist the referring clinician and the patient in determining the future course of action.
   f. *Category 5: Highly suggestive of malignancy; appropriate action should be taken.* This category is reserved for lesions that have a high probability of being malignant.

The terminology for mammography reporting has often been confusing. In an attempt to standardize breast imaging terminology, the American College of Radiology has developed a BIRADS breast imaging lexicon. The use of this reporting standard is encouraged to diminish the chance of potential misunderstandings in interpreting mammogram reports. The lexicon may be found in the BIRADS publication available from the American College of Radiology.

Screening Mammogram

Name of patient: _____

Patient's date of birth: _____

Name of referring clinician: _____

Type of examination (i.e., bilateral screening mammogram, right mammogram, left mammogram, diagnostic right/left mammogram)

Date of exam: _____

Clinical history: Screening exam. This examination is compared with the prior study of (date of prior study). There are scattered fibroglandular densities bilaterally (or other statements of breast composition according to the guidelines listed in item 2 above).

Impression: No change from the prior examination. No mammographic evidence of malignancy. Recommend continued yearly screening mammography (or recommendation for other imaging examination if a Category 0 is assigned).

BIRADS Category 1: Negative.

Breast Ultrasound

Clinical history: Give the indication for the exam, such as palpable mass, area of diffuse palpable nodularity, mammographic nodule, or mass.

Findings: Examination reveals no evidence for focal mass or cyst. Changes compatible with focal fibroglandular tissue are noted.

Impression: No ultrasound correlation to mammographic/palpable finding. (For exam because of palpable finding, "suggest clinical correlation.") (For exam because of mammographic finding, "mass on mammogram without ultrasound correlate. This, therefore, is compatible with normal fibroglandular tissue or an ultrasonographically occult mass. If the mass is new, then the decision for biopsy should be made.")

Stereotactically Guided Core Biopsy

Procedure: The _____ cm mass/calcifications in the _____ location of the (left or right) breast was identified. After explaining the procedure to the patient and obtaining informed consent, _____ passes with a _____ gage _____ needle was performed. Adequate samples were obtained. The patient tolerated the procedure well, without complications. Postprocedure instructions were reviewed with the patient.

Impression: Stereotactically guided _____ biopsy of (mass or calcifications) in the _____ location of the _____ breast. Samples were sent to Pathology.

Specimen Radiograph

Specimen radiography of the core biopsy specimens reveals mass/calcifications corresponding to mammographic findings. Samples were sent to Pathology in an annotated, alphanumeric grid, with the specimen radiograph.

Ultrasound-Guided Core Biopsy

Procedure: The _____ cm mass in the _____ location of the (left or right) breast was identified. After explaining the procedure to the patient and obtaining informed consent, _____ passes with an _____ gage _____ needle was performed. Adequate samples were obtained. The patient tolerated the procedure well, without complications. Postprocedure instructions were reviewed with the patient.

Impression: Ultrasound guided _____ biopsy of _____ cm mass in the _____ location of the _____ breast. Samples were sent to Pathology.

Preoperative Needle Localization

Procedure: After explaining the procedure to the patient and obtaining informed consent, a _____ cm (describe type of needle) needle and wire combination was placed in the (describe the type and location of the lesion). Methelene blue, 0.3 mL, was injected. The patient tolerated the procedure well, without complications. Annotated radiographs were sent to the operating room.

Impression: Preoperative needle localization of (describe the type and location of the lesion).

8 NUCLEAR MEDICINE

Ventilation and Perfusion (V/Q) Scan

Clinical history: Admitted after an episode of severe shortness of breath while walking two blocks.

Technique: The patient inhaled _____ mCi of (xenon-133 gas/xenon-127 gas/krypton-81 gas/aerosolized Tc-99m DTPA) for the ventilation phase images. The patient received an intravenous injection of _____ mCi of Tc-99-MAA for the perfusion phase images. This study was correlated with the chest X-ray dated _____.

Findings: There were no focal ventilatory defects in either lung. The right lung volume was slightly less than the left. There were no abnormal areas of retention. There were no vascular-appearing perfusion defects in either lung.

Interpretation: Given all of the above information, the above lung scan findings represent a low probability for pulmonary embolism as a cause for this patient's shortness of breath.

Whole-Body Bone Scan

Clinical history: Carcinoma of the breast, status post radiation therapy. Now with left-sided chest pain that radiates to the back. This study is compared with previous bone scan dated _____.

Technique: The patient received an intravenous injection of _____ mCi of Tc MDP. Whole body images were obtained with multiple spot views of the thorax, skull, and upper and lower extremities.

Findings: There are no abnormal areas of increased or decreased radiotracer activity. Both kidneys were visualized.

Interpretation: No evidence for metastatic bone disease.

Renal Transplant Scan

Clinical history: Status post renal transplantation from a living related donor (state date of transplant if known).

Technique/findings: The patient received an intravenous injection of _____ mCi of (Tc-99m MAG3/Tc-99m DTPA).

Flow phase of the study showed good blood flow to the transplant kidney in the left iliac fossa. In the image taken 2 min after injection, there was good initial uptake of the radiotracer by the kidney, which is uniformLy distributed by the renal parenchyma. Excretion was prompt, with the appearance of activity in the distal ureter at 3 min after injection. There were no abnormal extrarenal areas of increased or decreased radiotracer activity. There was no evidence of a dilated renal collecting system.

Interpretation: Good flow and function of the transplant kidney with no evidence of rejection.

Renal Captopril/Enalapril Scan

Clinical history: Hypertension that had been difficult to control. Admitted with elevated blood pressures, measured at 240 systolic over 120 diastolic in the coronary care unit. Multiple bruits on exam, including a questionable left renal bruit.

Technique: The patient received an intravenous injection of _____ mCi of Tc-99m DTPA for the pre-captopril (or pre-enalapril) renal scan. The patient returned and received a _____ mg dose of captopril (or enalapril) orally. Blood pressures were monitored for a period of 1 hour (or 15 min with enalapril), and the scan was repeated. The patient received an intravenous injection of _____ mCi of Tc-99m DTPA for the post-captopril (or -enalapril) images.

Findings: The pre-captopril (or enalapril) flow phase of the study showed good blood flow to the left kidney and fair blood flow to the right kidney. In the image taken 2 min after injection, there was good uptake of the radiotracer by both kidneys. In the images taken up to 30 min after injection, there was symmetric excretion of the radiotracer. The post-captopril (or -enalapril) renal scan demonstrated no significant differences in renal blood flow, uptake, or excretion of radiotracer.

Interpretation: No evidence of captopril (enalapril)-induced changes in renal function that would indicate physiologically significant renal artery stenosis.

Cardiac Perfusion Study

Clinical history: No previous cardiac history. Risk factors for coronary artery disease include hypertension, smoking, and family history.

Stress thallium SPECT: The patient received an intravenous injection of _____ mCi of (thallium 201-chloride/Tc-99m sestamibi/Tc-99m tetrofosmin). There were no abnormal areas of diminished perfusion on the tomographic images.

Stress physiology: The patient exercised for _____ min and _____ seconds on a Bruce protocol, achieving a peak heart rate of _____ and a peak blood pressure of _____ systolic. The test was terminated because of fatigue. There were no ischemic ST-T wave changes and no complaints of chest pain. The preexercise ECG showed normal sinus rhythm and nonspecific ST-T wave changes. The resting heart rate while standing was _____, with an associated blood pressure of _____.

Interpretation: Given all the above findings, there is no evidence for transient ischemia at this level of cardiac work.

Radionuclide Ventriculography

Clinical history: Myocardial infarction, (state date of MI). Coronary artery bypass graft surgery approximately _____ weeks prior to examination. Currently asymptomatic.

Techniques/findings: The patient received an intravenous injection of _____ mCi of (Tc-99m pertechnetate/Tc-99m HSA) (in vitro/in vivo/modified in vivo) labeled blood cells. A right ventricular first-pass study was performed. The right ventricle was normal in size, and function. The right ventricular ejection fraction was _____ %. The ventricles were imaged in the equilibrium state. The left ventricle was normal in size, and there were no wall motion abnormalities. The left ventricle ejection fraction was _____ %.

Interpretation: Normal global biventricular function at rest.

Hepatobiliary Scan

Clinical history: Increasing right upper quadrant pain.

Technique/findings: The patient received an intravenous injection of _____ μg/kg/min cholecystokinin before the intravenous administration of _____ mCi of (Tc-99m-mebrofenin/Tc-99m disofenin/Tc-99m lidofenin).

Blood flow images did not show any abnormal areas of increased hepatic blood flow.

In the image taken 2 min after injection, the radiotracer was uniformly distributed throughout the liver. There is prompt visualization of the gallbladder at 6 min after injection, with subsequent visualization of common bile duct and small bowel activity.

At 60 min after injection, the patient was given an intravenous infusion of _____ μg/kg/min of cholecystokinin by a mechanical pump over 3 min. Visually, there was rapid emptying of the gallbladder and probable enterogastric reflux. The measured ejection fraction was normal at _____ %.

Interpretation:

1. No evidence of cystic duct or common duct obstruction.
2. Normal gallbladder motor function.

GI Bleeding Scan

Clinical history: Episodic lower gastrointestinal bleeding.

Technique: The patient received an intravenous injection of _____ mCi of Tc-99m-pertechnetate (in vitro/in vivo/modified in vivo) labeled red blood cells.

Findings: Flow phase images centered over the abdomen did not show any abnormal areas of increased flow. Dynamic images taken every 2 min up to 2 h after injection did not show any abnormal areas of increased red blood cell activity.

Interpretation: No evidence of localizing source of gastrointestinal bleeding.

Gastric Emptying Scan

Clinical history: Severe reflux esophagitis.

Technique: The patient ate an entire meal of an egg sandwich labeled with _____ mCi of Tc-99m sulphur colloid. The quality control image did not show any retained radiotracer activity in the esophagus.

Findings: Visually, there was rapid emptying of the gastric contents with transit into the small bowel. The measure half-time for gastric emptying was _____ min (upper limits of normal $T_{1/2}$ = 105 ± 15 min).

Interpretation: No evidence of gastroparesis.

Thyroid Imaging

Clinical history: Primary hypothyroidism and secondary amenorrhea.

Technique: The patient received an oral dose of _____ μCi of (iodine-123/iodine-131/Tc-99m pertechnetate).

Findings: Both lobes of the thyroid gland appear normal in size. There was normal uptake of the radiotracer by the thyroid gland, with homogenous distribution, and no focal abnormalities. There was no evidence for ectopic thyroid tissue.

The 6-hour (or 24-hour) (iodine-123/iodine-131) uptake was within normal limits, measuring _____ % (normal range 10–30%).

Interpretation: Normal size and function of the thyroid gland, with no evidence of focal abnormality.

Regional Brain Perfusion Scan

Clinical history: One-week history of difficulty with speech.

Technique: The patient received an intravenous injection of _____ mCi of (Tc-99m HMPAO/iodine-123 IMP/Tc-99m ECD). Multiple transaxial, sagittal, and coronal views were obtained of cerebral perfusion.

Findings: There were no abnormal areas of increased or decreased perfusion.

Interpretation: No evidence of cerebral perfusion abnormality.

9 PEDIATRICS

Pediatric Chest Radiograph

Findings: The lungs are clear and well inflated. The cardiothymic silhouette is within normal limits. No bony abnormalities are seen.

Impression: Normal chest.

Pediatric Abdominal Radiograph

Findings: The bowel gas pattern is unremarkable, with no sign of abnormal distention or obstruction. No free air or air-fluid levels appear on this supine view. There is no evidence of organomegaly or abnormal calcifications. No bony abnormalities are seen.

Impression: Normal.

Pediatric Esophagram

Clinical history: Coughing with feeds.

Findings: The scout film of the chest is unremarkable. Oral and pharyngeal phases of swallow appeared normal with no misdirection of contrast into the nasal or tracheal airway. Normal esophageal peristalsis was seen, with no areas of narrowing. Intermittent observation during a period of quiet breathing showed no gastroesophageal reflux.

Impression: Normal esophagram.

Pediatric Upper GI

Clinical history: Three days of vomiting.

Findings: The scout film of the abdomen is unremarkable. Normal swallow is observed. The esophagus and stomach are unremarkable, with no obstruction to the gastric outlet. The duodenum, including the bulb, show normal configuration, with normal position of the ligament of Treitz. The initial loops of jejunum are normally positioned in the left upper quadrant. Throughout the exam, no gastroesophageal reflux was observed.

Impression: Normal upper GI.

Pediatric Barium Enema

Clinical history: Abdominal pain.

Findings: The scout film of the abdomen is unremarkable. Contrast was infused slowly by gravity, revealing normal configuration of the rectum, sigmoid, and proximal colon, with no evidence of malrotation or structure. The relative caliber of the rectum and sigmoid colon showed normal ratio. No significant reflux into the terminal ileum was obtained.

Impression: Normal single-contrast enema.

Air Enema for Intussusception Reduction

Clinical history: Suspected intussusception.

Technique/findings: After informed consent was obtained from the patient's parent, a rubber catheter was placed into the rectum, and air was gently insufflated by hand pressure. This filled a normal colon with no intraluminal filling defect to suggest the presence of intussusception. There was reflux of air into the terminal ileum and distention of small bowel.

Impression: No evidence of intussusception by air enema.

Voiding Cystourethrogram

Clinical history: Repeated urinary tract infections.

Technique/findings: The scout film of the abdomen shows no bony or soft tissue abnormality. The bladder was catheterized with a _____ tube, and _____ mL of residual urine was removed. The bladder was then filled with _____ mL of Cysto-Conray. The outline of the filled bladder is unremarkable. There was no vesicoureteral reflux during the filling or voiding phases. Voiding revealed a normal urethra and no postvoid residual.

Impression: Normal voiding cystourethrogram.

Baby Head Ultrasound

Clinical history: Two-day-old, formerly 32-week gestation.

Findings: The ventricles are normal in caliber and configuration. There are no midline anomalies. There is no evidence of intraventricular or parenchymal hemorrhage.

Impression: Normal head ultrasound.

Renal and Bladder Ultrasound

Clinical history: Hydronephrosis on prenatal ultrasound.

Findings: The right kidney measures _____ cm in length, and the left kidney measures _____ cm. There is no evidence of hydronephrosis, hydroureter, or stones. Renal echogenicity is normal. The filled bladder contains _____ mL of urine and shows no debris or stones. Wall thickness is normal. There is no postvoid residual.

Impression: Normal renal and bladder ultrasound.

Hip Ultrasound

Clinical history: Infant with hip "click" on physical examination.

Technique/findings: Views were taken in the coronal and transverse orientation. The hip joints demonstrate normal articulation. The femoral heads measure _____ cm in diameter bilaterally. Alpha angles measure_____ degrees bilaterally, and beta angles measure _____ degrees bilaterally. There is no effusion. Stress views demonstrate no subluxation of the femoral heads.

Impression: Normal hip ultrasound.

Bone Age

Clinical history: Precocious puberty.

Findings: The patient's chronologic age is _____ years and _____ months. The bone age is most consistent with that of a male/female of _____ years and _____ months of age.

Impression: Bone age in concordance with chronologic age.

10 ANGIOGRAPHY

Aortogram with Runoff

Clinical history: Claudication.

Preprocedure diagnosis: Atherosclerosis.

Postprocedure diagnosis: Diffuse atherosclerosis without vascular obstruction.

Procedure: Aortogram with runoff

Physicians: Dr. _____ and Dr. _____ .

Contrast: Visipaque 320, 250 mL.

Medications: 1 mg midazolam and 50 µg Fentanyl iv.

Complications: None.

Procedure/findings: The procedure, risks, and options were discussed with the patient, who gave written consent for the procedure and agreed to proceed. The groins were sterilely prepped and draped bilaterally. Under local anesthesia (_____ mL 1.5% lidocaine), the right common femoral artery was punctured using an 18-g Potts needle. A 5-Fr sheath was placed and a 5-Fr pigtail catheter was advanced into the abdominal aorta over an 0.035-inch Bentson guidewire and placed at the level of the renal arteries. The pigtail catheter was used to perform a digital subtraction aortogram, both oblique views of the pelvis and a standard long film runoff series. After the aortogram and oblique pelvic views, the catheter was repositioned and placed into each external iliac artery before obtaining the standard extremity runoff views. Digital subtraction views of the feet were also performed.

There was minimal atherosclerotic disease of the abdominal aorta and the common iliac arteries. Single renal arteries were noted bilaterally. The internal and external iliac arteries were patent but demonstrated minimal atherosclerotic disease, as did the common femoral, superficial femoral, profunda femoris, popliteal, anterior tibial, posterior tibial, and peroneal arteries. The anterior tibial, posterior tibial, and peroneal arteries were patent to the level of the foot. The dorsalis pedis arteries also demonstrated minimal atherosclerotic disease but were patent.

Interpretation/conclusion: Diffuse mild atherosclerotic disease without vessel occlusion.

Disposition: The patient returned to the recovery room in good condition and will be monitored for 6 h before reassessment and possibly discharged at that time.

8 General Requirements and Policies

1 REQUIREMENTS FOR AMERICAN BOARD OF RADIOLOGY ELIGIBILITY

During the course of their postdoctoral training, residents are expected to fulfill the requirements to be eligible to take the American Board of Radiology (ABR) written and oral examinations in their fourth year. These requirements are as follows:

1. Candidates beginning their graduate medical education after January 1, 1997 will be required to have 5 years of approved training with a minimum of 4 years in diagnostic radiology. These 4 years of diagnostic training must be spent in a department approved for training in diagnostic radiology by the Residency Review Committee (RRC) for diagnostic radiology of the Accreditation Council for Graduate Medical Education (ACGME) or by the Royal College of Physicians and Surgeons of Canada (RCPSC). A minimum of 6 months but no more than 12 months must be spent in Nuclear Radiology in the 4-year diagnostic training program.

2. The remaining year of training must be in an ACGME-approved clinical training program such as internal medicine, pediatrics, surgery or surgical specialties, OB/GYN, neurology, family practice, emergency medicine, or any combination of these. The clinical year will usually be the first year of postgraduate training. No more than 3 months can be in radiology, radiation oncology, or pathology. All clinical training must be in an ACGME, RCPSC, American Osteopathic Association, or equivalent approved training program.

3. It is not the intent of the ABR for programs to use any of the 4 years of radiology training for traditional fellowship training.

The designation "fellowship" is reserved for training beyond the 4-year diagnostic radiology training residency.

4. In a 4-year approved diagnostic radiology residency program, not more than 12 months of the required 48 months of training can be spent in any single discipline. (Research is considered a discipline.)

5. In a 4-year diagnostic program, the resident is expected to remain in that program for all 4 years. If a transfer to another program is desired, that transfer must have verification from the initial program director that the resident has successfully completed the training in their institution with a listing of specific rotations. This training must be accepted by the new program director. If a program director states that a resident has not successfully completed training in that program, this statement must have the signatures of two other faculty members from the same program supporting the unsatisfactory completion of the previous program.

6. Candidates will be considered for the physics portion of the written examination only when they have completed 12 months of diagnostic radiology training. After 24 months of radiology training, candidates will be allowed to sit for the clinical portion of the written examination.

7. Residents must have basic life support certification. Advanced Cardiac Life Support certification is encouraged.

8. Program directors will be asked to verify only months of training for resident in their program. They will not be asked to attest to the residents' professional qualifications until the residents' fourth year, prior to the oral examination. A complete report of all residents will be sent to the program directors with details for their internal use only.

9. Within the required period(s) of training, the total such leave and vacation time may not exceed 6 calendar weeks (30 working days) for fellows in a 1-year program, 12 calendar weeks (60 working days) for residents in a 2-year program, 18 calendar weeks (90 working days) for residents in a 3-year program, and 24 calendar weeks (120 working days) for residents in a 4-year program. If a longer leave of absence is granted, the required period of graduate medical education must be extended accordingly.

Holman Research Pathway

The ABR Holman Research Pathway is an integrated program that combines training in research with training in clinical radiology. This pathway is recommended only for physicians who are planning a career that focuses primarily on basic science or clinical research. Other physicians should pursue the standard 5 years of training. Prior board approval must be obtained before undertaking the ABR research pathway. This program is designed for the exceptional trainee, and entry implies a commitment to its completion and a research career.

Requirements for ABR Eligibility/Credit: *International Medical Graduates*

The following guidelines are used for granting credit to diagnostic radiologists trained outside the United States or Canada.

Any exceptions to the guidelines must have approval of the Executive Committee of the ABR.

1. Individuals from accredited training programs and with a confirmed fellowship in the following will receive 2 years' credit. (Individuals who have completed 4 years of training in diagnostic radiology in the United Kingdom, but without a fellowship, will receive 1 year of credit, requiring 3 additional years of residency training at one institution.)
   a. The Royal College of Radiologists, London
   b. The Royal Australasian College of Radiologists
   c. Faculty of Radiologists, Royal College of Surgeons, Ireland
   d. Faculty of Radiology, The College of Medicine of South Africa.

2. In addition to the above, to be admitted to the ABR certifying examination, candidates must also:
   a. Complete 2 years of residency training in an ACGME-approved program, *or*
   b. Complete 1 year of residency training and 1 year of fellowship training in an ACGME-approved program. Only 1 year of fellowship training will be allowed, and no further training in the discipline of the fellowship is allowed.
   c. Complete 2 full-time clinical years on the faculty in a radiology department at one institution that offers an ACGME-approved residency in diagnostic radiology (request for credit must be initiated by the Department Chair with letters of recommendation from two other full-time clinical staff members), *or*
   d. Complete a combination of 1-year residency (or fellowship) and 1-year full-time staff service.

3. For all other international training, no credit will be allowed toward accrual for the 4 years required to take the ABR exams.

4. Only 1 year of credit will be allowed to individuals for US/Canada fellowships taken in Departments of Radiology with ACGME-approved residencies. Upon granting a year of credit, if in a single discipline, i.e., neuroradiology or nuclear medicine, no further training will be allowed in that discipline during the 3-year residency fulfillment.

5. Individuals serving 4 continuous years at one institution (as a full-time clinical faculty member in a Department of Radiology with an ACGME/RCPSC-approved program) will be considered for the ABR examination. Prior to consideration, written request of the individual and the Department Chair is required, along with letters of support from two other members of the clinical faculty. These individuals must provide validation of a clinical year and have passed the entire United States Medical Licensing Examination (USMLE).

6. An approved clinical year is required. Credit will be given for a clinical year in Canada, Australia, England, Hong Kong, Ireland, Scotland, or South Africa only.

OTHER GUIDELINES

1. Training or experience is the main justification for granting credit. Requests for credit should be submitted in writing to the Executive Director of the ABR. Although letters of recommendation are helpful, they alone will not result in allowing an individual to take the examination.

2. Official credit for fulfillment of the individual's residency requirement will be given only at the request of a Program Director. The Program Director must accept any credit given as part of that residency program.

3. Nuclear Radiology training (6 months) must be verified for all candidates irrespective of the mechanism used for granting of credit.

2 BOARD EXAMINATIONS

Diagnostic Radiology

Radiology residents and other candidates must pass both a written and an oral examination to be certified by the ABR. The physics portion of the written examination can be taken as early as the second year of radiology residency, and the clinical portion of the written examination can be taken beginning in the third year of residency. The oral portion of the board certification is taken in the final year of residency training prior to completion of the residency program. Residents will be notified of upcoming board examination dates and deadlines well in advance. Specific questions should be directed to the Resident Secretary, or the Residency Director.

Both the physics exam and the written clinical exam are 1-day tests usually taken in September. Past residents have done very well preparing for the written boards by concentrating on other residents' notes and old test questions. Residents taking the written exam should start asking residents who have completed the written examination(s) for access to their notes by January. Looking at notes more than 5 years old is probably not an effective use of time. Some residents also use the American College of Radiology (ACR) syllabi for studying. The "classic" major texts are essential reading as well. Results of the written boards take approximately 6 weeks to receive.

Residents may take the physics portion of the written boards as a separate exam, in the beginning of the second year of residency. Interested residents need to apply early to be eligible for the physics exam. Candidates must pass both portions of the written boards to qualify for the oral boards. Candidates who fail the diagnostic portion of the written boards will be rescheduled for the following year. Candidates who fail the physics portion only can retake it in the early part of the following year; upon passing, they can still qualify for the oral boards that year.

Oral boards are taken during the early summer, at the end of the fourth year of residency training. The oral board is a half-day test. Candidates are tested for 25 minutes in each of 10 areas: Chest, Orthopedics, GI, Genitourinary, Ultrasound, Neuroradiology, Mammography, Cardiac/Interventional, Pediatrics, and Nuclear Medicine. The intention of the oral boards is to imitate, to the extent possible, real-life consultations between a radiologist (the candidate) and a referring physician (the examiner). Emphasis is placed on the ability to interpret images and express clearly and succinctly what the images disclose. Every effort is made to show the candidate as many cases as possible in each 25-minute period. The candidate is expected to analyze the images accurately, make a diagnosis, and state a reasonable differential. Lengthy questioning about each case and protracted discussion are usually avoided. The board is looking for candidates who can recognize abnormalities and express in appropriately measured phrases what is seen and what it means.

The best way to study for the oral boards is to see as many real-life cases as possible during the entire residency training, to read extensively, starting from year one, and to attend conferences and lectures regularly. No amount of "cramming" in the fourth year of training can make up for 3 years of neglect. Oral Board results take approximately 7–10 days to receive. A candidate who fails the oral boards may be reexamined in 1 year. A new fee is required. Three consecutive oral failures requires an applicant to retake the entire written boards examination, including the physics section. Failure to accept an appointment, cancel an appointment, or appear for an appointment constitutes a failure. Candidates can conditionally pass the exam, with repeat exams required in one, two, or three of the clinical areas. This secondary exam is usually given in the beginning of November, the same year.

Application for the Exam

Application for examination must be made in exact duplicate (two original copies on prescribed forms, which may be obtained from the ABR office). No Xerox or any other kind of copy will be accepted. These forms must be forwarded by the deadline of September 30, together with:

- Three recent passport-type photographs (no larger than 3 × 3 inches) autographed on the front (informal Polaroid or other snapshots are *not* acceptable); the Program Director must countersign photos (also on the front) attesting to validity; the application cannot be accepted without fulfillment of this requirement, *and*

- Current application fee (in U.S. currency)

Current applications must be postmarked by September 30 for registration in the next year's written examination. There is a nonrefundable penalty fee of $200 for any application postmarked between October 1 and October 31. No applications will be accepted after October 31 for examination in that year. All returned checks and declined credit cards will be subject to a $100 processing fee. Incomplete applications will not be accepted. The postmark affixed to the last item received to complete the application must be on or before the deadline date. All applications must be typed or neatly printed (in ink). In the event of withdrawal of an application, a portion of the fee may be refunded. An administrative fee will be retained.

A candidate who finds it necessary for any reason to cancel at least 20 days prior to the first day of the examination after acceptance of an appointment for either the written or oral examination shall be required to submit an additional fee. This fee represents administrative costs to the Board. A candidate who fails to appear for an examination without notifying the office of the ABR at least 20 days prior to the first date of the examination will be charged the full application fee.

Examination Fees

APPLICATION FEE

Written exam fee	$600
Oral exam fee	$600
Administration fee	$600 (due upon submission of application prior to Sept. 30)
Late filing fee	$200
Reexamination fee	$750
Cancellation fee	$200 (20 days before exam)
	$1,800 (less than 20 days)

Contact Information

The American Board of Radiology
5255 East Williams Circle, Suite 3200
Tucson, AZ 85711
Phone: (520) 790-2900
Fax: (520) 790-3200
E-mail: info@theabr.org

Preparation for the ABR Exam

Results of a recent survey of 100 successful first-time takers of the boards were summarized in the *ABR Examiner* 1:3. Seven questions were asked, which are given below with comments.

1. What helped you most in preparing for the exam?

    Specific suggestions included participating in twice-daily board review conferences held for several months in spring and summer, studying old questions (written exam), studying ACR video disks, and mock board sessions (oral exam). ACR files were also felt to be helpful, but many were said to be outdated. One successful candidate offered that the GI, Genitourimary, Bone and Pediatric sections of the film library were best. The ACR disks were said to be best for GI, Genitourimary, Neuroradiology, Pediatric Radiology, Bone, and Ultrasound. The real-time video displays on the ACR ultrasound disk were particularly helpful since this format is used at the boards. The ACR syllabi were thought to be quite good, but one successful candidate found they took up too much time. Reviewing them earlier in residency was advised.

2. What that you read was especially helpful?

    The ACR film library (Learning File) and the ACR video discs were specifically cited as helpful. Textbooks assigned for each month of rotation were thought to be especially valuable.

Dahnert's radiology review was a helpful supplement to textbooks. Many mentioned reviewing an anatomy text and Armed Forces Institute of Pathology (AFIP) notes. For the oral examination, radiology review course syllabi and selected textbooks were cited.

3. If you attended a review course, was it helpful? In what way?

    Around half of those replying attended a review course, and most thought it was very good. Most said the course provided reassurance and a passive respite from the active studying experience. Others declined to attend such a course, believing that the best review is the AFIP, or better yet, organized personal review after paying attention for 4 years.

4. How helpful were mock boards?

    Everyone thought that mock boards were very helpful. Particularly valuable were sessions conducted by senior faculty and by guest examiners on the real boards who simulated actual test conditions. Mock boards provided an opportunity to hear oneself and others articulate in a structured environment. That enabled the participants to realize what differentials were difficult and needed polishing.

5. What would you have done differently in preparing for or taking the examination?

    Some offered advice to concentrate on learning reasonable differential diagnoses earlier in the residency and to keep learning esoteric facts to a minimum. Everyone recommended studying hard for the physics.

6. Were you as schizophrenic in your senior year as some program directors tell us many of their residents are? What do you feel would help to reduce the madness?

    Most thought there was nothing that could be done about the board paranoia. Some thought it had more to do with the obsessive/compulsive personality types that are attracted to medicine. The horror stories about excellent resident conditioning and examiners that may rake you over the coals were enough to scare some candidates. Putting a stop to such horror stories was mentioned as an important element in reducing the tension associated with the examination. Pressure on the candidates is great because the stakes are very high on this examination, cited some of the respondents. With the tightening of the job market, board certification is becoming a necessity. Most successful candidates agreed that the best way to reduce the anxiety associated with the examination is a steady pace of reading, conference attendance, and so on over the 4 years, and not waiting until the last few weeks or months to cram for the examination.

7. What advice would you offer to those preparing for the written or oral examination?

    Most of the advice regarding the written examination consisted of suggestions that the candidates study hard for physics and study old test questions. For the oral examination, most of the respondents commented that they were overprepared and that they learned more by applying themselves evenly during the 4 years of training than they did by cramming at the end. Several recognized that the day-to-day experience of interpreting films was probably the best preparation for the oral boards. Several persons offered the same advice: go to a good program, read seriously and industriously for 4 years, and be attentive every day to the variety of patients and pathology you encounter. Go to all available conferences, attend all available readout sessions, and ask questions constantly. Take good notes in conference and at the viewbox (a great way to review later). Attend board review sessions for senior residents. Trying to cram it all into the last year was specifically cited as counterproductive.

Test Results

Since the introduction of the new testing policy for the ABR physics exam in 1998, the pass rates for second-year resident first-time takers averaged approximately 85%. The pass rate for third-year residents taking the physics exam for the first time was approximately 91%. The third-year residents taking only the clinical portion of the exam had an average pass rate of approximately 85% and a fail rate of approximately 15%. The pass rate for third-year residents taking both the physics and clinical portions of the exam averaged approximately 63% (condition rates approximately 11%; fail rates approximately 26%).

First-time fourth-year residents taking only the physics exam had a pass rate of 100% in 1999. (There were only three individuals in this category during the 1999 testing.) During the same year, fourth-year residents taking only the clinical portion of the exam managed a 96% pass rate (4% fail rate). The fourth-year residents taking only the clinical portion of the exam had a 97% pass rate and a 3% fail rate in 2000. During this same year the pass rate was 27% for all first-time takers (30% condition rate; 27% fail rate).

From 1995 to 1998, the pass rate for the diagnostic written examination for first-time takers has averaged approximately 91%, with a 5% fail rate and a 4% condition rate. During this same period, repeat examinees did not fare nearly as well with pass rates averaging approximately 35% (condition rates approximately 8%; fail rates approximately 57%). From 1999 to 2000, fourth-year residents taking the clinical portion of the diagnostic written exam had pass rates averaging 97%, and a fail rate of 3%. Comparatively, all first-time takers of both the diagnostic written and physics exam had an average pass rate of 56%, a condition rate of 16%, and a fail rate of 28%. Individuals repeating the diagnostic written examination from 1999 to 2000 had pass, condition, and fail rates of 35, 5, and 60%, respectively.

Since the mid-1990s, examinees taking the oral exam for the first time have had a pass rate of approximately 78%. This average is up substantially from the 1995 pass rate of 69%. The rate of first-time takers conditioning the exam has also decreased from 27% in 1995 and has averaged approximately 16–17% since that time. The fail rate for the first-time takers has remained stable at approximately 3–5%. Examinees repeating the oral examination had a dramatically lower average pass rate of approximately 27% and correspondingly higher rates of conditioning and failure averaging 32 and 41%, respectively.

Note: The statistics above reflect the cumulative averages during the time periods specifically stated. The most recent statistics are based on the latest information that had been released by the ABR at the time the book went to press.

Certificates of Added Qualification/ Special Competence

In 1995, the ABR established certificates of added qualifications (CAQs) in Pediatric Radiology, Vascular/Interventional Radiology, and Neuroradiology. This was done to gain recognition by the American Board of Medical Specialties (ABMS) that these already established subspecialty areas are within the domain of radiology and to provide a certification examination for individuals completing fellowships already approved by the ACGME. The CAQs must be renewed every 10 years because of the ABMS requirement for time limits to be placed on all new certificates. Completion of a 1-year fellowship in Neuroradiology, Pediatric Radiology, or Vascular/Interventional Radiology is also necessary to be eligible for taking a CAQ exam. Exceptions were initially made for practicing physicians without fellowship training who met various practice criteria to be eligible to take a CAQ exam. These exceptions are no longer applicable, and all candidates seeking a CAQ must now have completed an accredited fellowship and have the other necessary training requirements (see below). The other criteria (i.e., number of procedures performed) for eligibility have been determined specifically for each of the three separate subspecialties. Further information and an application for a CAQ exam can be obtained by contacting the ABR.

A Certificate of Diagnostic Radiology with Special Competence in Nuclear Radiology is also available to Diplomates of the ABR. Similar to the CAQ examinations, the oral exam in Nuclear Radiology is offered annually, and successful candidates will be offered a 10-year certificate in Diagnostic Radiology with Special Competence in Nuclear Radiology.

Examination Dates, Application, and Fees

EXAMINATION DATES

The oral examinations for Neuroradiology, Nuclear Radiology, Pediatric Radiology, and Vascular and Interventional Radiology are usually offered at the same time in early November. The examination fees are currently identical for all four examinations ($1,200), as are the reexamination fees ($600).

APPLICATION

Application for examination must be made in exact duplicate (two original copies on prescribed forms obtained through the ABR office). No copies of the forms will be accepted. These forms must be forwarded by the deadline of April 31, together with:

1. Two recent passport-type photographs (no larger than 3 × 3 inches) signed on the front. (Informal photographs are not acceptable.) The application cannot be accepted without fulfillment of this requirement, *and*
2. Current application fee (US currency).

The check should be made payable to The American Board of Radiology, Inc.

Incomplete applications will not be accepted. The postmark affixed to the last item received to complete the application must be on or before the deadline date.

There is a nonrefundable penalty fee of $200 for any applications postmarked between May 1 and May 31. No applications will be accepted after May 31 for the examination in that year.

All returned checks and declined credit cards will be subject to a $100 processing fee.

In the event of withdrawal of an application, a portion of the fee may be refunded. An administrative fee will be retained.

Training Requirements

Neuroradiology: Candidates must successfully complete 1 year of fellowship training (after residency) in a Neuroradiology Program approved for such training and accredited by the ACGME and 1 year of practice or additional approved training (one-third of that time) in Neuroradiology. The successful completion of fellowship training must be documented in a letter from the Program Director. The candidates' practice experience must be verified in a letter from the Chief of Service or Department Chairman.

Nuclear Radiology: Candidates must successfully complete 1 year of fellowship training (after residency) in a Nuclear Radiology Program approved for such training by the Residency Review Committee (RRC) for Diagnostic Radiology or in a department approved for training in Nuclear Medicine by the RRC for Nuclear Medicine and accredited by the ACGME. No credit will be given for any nuclear training obtained during the 4 years of Diagnostic Radiology.

Pediatric Radiology: Candidates must successfully complete 1 year of fellowship training (after residency) in a Pediatric Radiology Program approved for such training and accredited by the ACGME. Candidates must also have 1 year of practice or additional approved training (one-third of that time) in Pediatric Radiology. Fellowship training must be documented in a letter from the Program Director. The candidates' practice experience must be verified in a letter from the Chief of Service or Department Chairman.

Vascular and Interventional Radiology: Candidates must successfully complete 1 year of fellowship training (after residency) in a Vascular and Interventional Program approved for such training and accredited by the ACGME and have 1 year of practice or additional approved training (one-third of that time) in Vascular and Interventional Radiology. Successful completion of fellowship training must be documented in a letter from the Program Director. The candidates' practice experience must be verified in a letter from the Chief of Service or Department Chairman.

To qualify for the examination, all candidates must present documentation of having completed at least 500 invasive cases (prime operator in at least 50%) with diverse experience in vascular and nonvascular interventions. These cases must include a minimum of 100 angiograms, 25 angioplasties, and 15 percutaneous renal procedures. The log must be verified and signed by the Chief of the Radiology Service and Chief of the Medical Staff.

Additional Information

Specific information regarding the examinations, reexaminations, pass rates, fees, deadlines, leaves of absence and other items can be obtained directly from the ABR (*see* Section 2 for contact information).

FELLOWSHIPS

During the late 1990s and in the early part of the first decade of the new millennium, approximately 70–80% of radiology residents have elected to pursue additional training in a fellowship program. Whether or not to do a fellowship is a personal decision, as is the field in which to pursue the fellowship. Fellowships are available in most radiology specialties, and some programs offer combined fellowships. To make fellowship selection somewhat easier, the ACR publishes a directory of fellowship programs. Fellowship advertisements can also be found in the back of the journals (*Radiology* and the *American Journal of Roentgenology*).

Applications are usually accepted during the fall of your third year, and the interviews will follow the application process.

NEURORADIOLOGY FELLOWSHIP APPLICATION MATCH PROGRAM

Administered by the National Residency Match Program (NRMP), the Neuroradiology Fellowship Application Match Program was formed to direct the selection of fellowship candidates for this subspecialty. The candidates beginning their fellowship on July 1, 2002 were the first to be affected by this new progam.

Nearly all the 96 fellowship programs in the United States and Canada participated in the first Neuroradiology Fellowship Match. All candidates applying for fellowship training in Neuroradiology (with the exception of internal candidates and candidates in combined Interventional/Neuroradiology Programs) should plan to submit a match application as long as this matching program exists.

Program application documents are usually available in mid-September, and the deadline for participation is early November. The interview season begins in mid-October, and the rankings for the candidates are due in late December. Match day is held separately from the traditional residency match, usually in mid-January.

The NRMP fellowship match for Neuroradiology is supported by the American Society of Neuroradiology (ASNR). The ASNR has expressed hope that this process will improve the fellowship selection procedure by making the process more organized and systematic. The Association of Program Directors in Diagnostic Radiology (APDR) has also expressed support for this matching process and is an advocate for the implementation of a universal fellowship application form, which would allow the other subspecialty fellowship programs to be joined into a single matching program. At the time the book went to press, discussions were underway to establish a single-match process for all radiology fellowships. Additional information about the Neuroradiology Fellowship Application Match Program can be found at the ASNR web site (www.asnr.org).

BOARD REVIEW COURSES

Many institutions offer review courses for Radiology residents. Several of these courses are specifically intended to prepare residents for boards. The most well-known radiology course is a radiology/pathology correlation and review given by the AFIP and is usually attended by residents in their third year of training. Popular review courses designed for board preparation include the Duke Review Course and the University of San Diego Review Course, both given in the spring.

USMLE PART 3

Completion of the USMLE is required before gaining a medical license in the state of your residency. Completion of USMLE Step 3 early in your residency is recommended for many reasons. The examination format and content is similar to that of Step 2, testing general medical clinical understanding and the application of your knowledge in unsupervised settings. As you turn your focus to studying radiology during internship or residency, taking time to prepare for Step 3 becomes an increasing burden the longer you wait. Furthermore, your memory of the general medical knowledge gained in medical school and internship will undoubtedly diminish proportionate to your time into residency. This may not necessarily jeopardize the outcome of your test (pass versus fail), but it may increase your level of anxiety for taking the test and contribute to a more thorough preparation that would not be required earlier in training. Once you have passed all three steps, you are eligible for state licensure (after fulfilling other requirements such as time in postdoctorate training, which varies by state). Moonlighting opportunities then become an option for augmenting your income after licensure.

The exam is offered in June and December each year. If your training program does not provide application materials, contact your state licensing board of the Federation of State Medical Boards (FSMB) directly for information.

FSMB
6000 Western Place, Suite 707
Fort Worth, TX 76107
(817) 735-0722

3 EXAMPLES OF LEAVE POLICY

Maternity Leave

After an uncomplicated pregnancy, residents may receive a total of 6 weeks of leave. Salary will be provided and paid by the usual source. Residents should request leave by submitting written notification to the Program Director and by notifying the chief resident as soon as possible (first trimester). Five weeks will be designated as sick leave and 1 week as paid parental leave. A complicated pregnancy will be handled through sick leave and disability policies. If a resident who has taken maternity leave is unable to fulfill the requirements for board eligibility within the standard training period, then vacation time may be used to meet the requirements. If the available vacation time is not adequate to fulfill the requirements, then an extended appointment period beyond the usual 4 years, with salary and benefits, will be granted, provided the resident has not exceeded the usual 6-week maternity leave and has utilized all available vacation time for maternity leave. If the resident wishes to prolong maternity leave for nonmedical reasons, this must be negotiated with the Program Director and would require an interruption in appointment (resignation) without pay. Benefits during this time may be purchased through the institution and are the responsibility of the resident. Reinstatement into the program depends on availability of positions and cannot be guaranteed for voluntary interruption of appointment.

Adoption Leave

After the adoption of a child, a parent who is the primary caregiver for a child will be given a 6-week leave with pay. Five weeks are designated as adoption leave and 1 week as paid parental leave. If both parents are housestaff or fellows, only the parent who is the primary caregiver will be given the 6-week leave. The other parent is eligible for 1 week of paid parental leave (see below). Residents are expected to notify the chief resident as soon as they realize they need adoption leave, so that scheduling changes can be made.

Parental Leave

After the birth or adoption of a child, a parent may receive up to 1 week of paid leave. Residents are expected to notify their chief resident as soon as they realize they will need parental leave, so that scheduling changes can be made.

Illness

A maximum of 13 consecutive weeks of paid leave for medical reasons may be granted to housestaff, with the approval of the Program Director and the appropriate representative from the school of medicine. After 90 consecutive days of illness, housestaff must apply for benefits under the institution's disability plan. This policy also applies to extended leave after a complicated pregnancy.

The amount of leave taken may affect the resident's ability to meet requirements for board eligibility. According to ABR guidelines, a candidate is eligible for board certification within the standard training period of 4 years if they have missed less than:

12 weeks or 60 days in a 2-year period
18 weeks or 90 days in a 3-year period
24 weeks or 120 days in a 4-year period

Vacation time may be utilized to ensure completion of training requirements within the standard training period.

4 PROCEDURE LOGS

Residents should keep a log of the procedures they have done. These logs will give prospective employers some information regarding your previous experience, are necessary to satisfy certain accreditation program requirements, and may be helpful in obtaining hospital privileges during the credentialing process. Each entry should include patient identification number, the procedure, the primary and secondary physicians, and the outcome. Residents should also compile a list of interesting cases. This list is especially useful when preparing case conferences and lectures.

5 ARMED FORCES INSTITUTE OF PATHOLOGY (AFIP)

This rotation at the AFIP in Washington, DC is an intensive 6-week learning experience where residents will hear some of the best lectures ever given on radiologic-pathologic correlation. The AFIP requires each resident to prepare and present two outstanding cases with radiology-pathology correlation, for admission to the course. Submission forms are available on the internet (http://www.afip.mil/). Residents should obtain these forms and complete them before the first day of their AFIP rotation. Cases should have excellent gross photos as well as radiology.

A rare case does not necessarily constitute a good AFIP case. The Institute is interested in cases that correlate the radiology with the pathology, and some of the best examples have been of classic cases of more common disease such as fibrous dysplasia or Crohn's disease. A rare "amazingoma" with a so-so MRI and poor gross photos is not considered a good case. You should start looking for good cases in your second year of residency (or even sooner).

Location

The AFIP and the Radiologic Pathology Education Center are located on the campus of Walter Reed Army Medical Center in northwest Washington, DC, near both Silver Spring and Tacoma Park Metro stations (red line).

Parking

All-day street parking is extremely limited in the area around the AFIP, and the use of public transportation is encouraged.

Housing

The packet of information provided by the AFIP has limited information on housing in the area. Consultation with a fellow resident who has attended the course or your Radiology Department is recommended. Housing close to public transportation is a prime consideration. Contact the course coordinators with any questions.

More on Cases

The two most important parameters used to evaluate a case are:

1. Excellence of correlative gross photography
2. Completeness and quality of the radiologic images.

The AFIP course coordinators state that the cases resulting in the best radiologic-pathologic correlation result from a resident's personal involvement in obtaining gross photographs of the resected specimen or autopsy. This can be accomplished during a rotation when a patient with interesting radiologic findings has a lesion removed or if an autopsy is performed. This can be discovered during your interaction with the consulting clinicians, and plans can subsequently be made for photographing the specimen after surgery or during autopsy. A second method is to start with cases that already have the gross photographs (by consultation with your pathologists or surgeons). If you have any questions about the suitability of your case, contact the case manager before you prepare the case. Requirements for AFIP cases include pertinent radiologic images (originals), color photography of the gross pathology, pathologic material (slides), and clinical data (discharge summary, operative report, radiologic reports, pertinent lab data, physiologic data, and so on). Additional paperwork provided in the AFIP packet must be completed for each case. Useful numbers are as follows:

Course Coordinators (202) 782-2272/2270
Case Coordinators (202) 782-2172/2170
Metro information (202) 637-7000
Washington, DC information (202) 724-4091

More detailed information and instructions for the course are provided in the AFIP packet, but the discussion above should prove useful in preliminary planning of cases and travel to the course.

6 SAMPLE RESIDENCY CURRICULUM (WITH NIGHT FLOAT SYSTEM)

First Year

Service	Weeks
General	10–12
GI/Genitourinary	8–10
Emergency Room	8–10
Musculoskeletal	4
CT	3
Neuroradiology	3
Ultrasound	3
Nuclear Medicine	4
Orientation	1

Second Year

Service	Weeks
Interventional Radiology	6
CT	6–8
Neuroradiology	5–6
Nuclear Medicine	4–8
Nights	7–8
General	6–8
Pediatrics	0–4
Mammography	3

Third Year

Service	Weeks
Ultrasound	6–8
AFIP	6
Nights	7–8
General	4–6
Nuclear Medicine	4–8
Body MRI	6
Pediatrics	2–6
Interventional Radiology	4
Musculoskeletal	4

Fourth Year

Service	Weeks
Interventional Radiology	4
Neuroradiology	3
Ultrasound	3
CT	3
Nuclear Medicine	4–6
Pediatrics	3
Mammography	3
GI/Genitourinary	2–3
Elective	12

Fellowship

A general guideline for fellowships is that subspecialty training in radiology is to commence after the completion of a 5-year residency program. According to the ABR, Fellowship curricula will vary dramatically according to the subspecialty, type of practice, available equipment and a host of other factors. It is not the intent of the ABR that programs should use any of the 4 years of training in diagnostic radiology for traditional fellowship training.

7 MEETING/EDUCATIONAL TIMELINE

The following list is not meant to be exhaustive or all inclusive. It is, however, an index of some of the more popular radiologic and general medical meetings and a time-focused listing of some of the important educational deadlines.

January

ACNP (American College of Nuclear Physicians) Meeting

February

Inservice Exam (first-, second-, third-year residents)

Application deadline, USMLE Exam (June)

SGR (Society of Gastrointestinal Radiologists) Meeting

ACGME (Accreditation Council for Graduate Medical Education) Meeting

March

SCVIR (Society of Cardiovascular and Interventional Radiology) Meeting

AVIR (Association of Vascular and Interventional Radiographers) Meeting

STR (Society of Thoracic Radiology) Meeting

ASTRO (American Society for Therapeutic Radiology and Oncology) Meeting

ECR (European Congress of Radiology)

SSR (Society of Skeletal Radiology)

SUR (Society of Uroradiology)

RRC (Residency Review Committee) Meeting, Diagnostic Radiology

April

Association of University Radiologists (AUR) Meeting

A³CR² (American Association of Academic Chief Residents in Radiology) Meeting; held in Conjunction with the AUR

SCARD (Society of Chairmen of Academic Radiology Departments) Meeting

SCBT/MR (Society of Computed Body Tomography and Magnetic Resonance) Meeting

ASHNR (American Society of Head and Neck Radiology) Meeting

ASER (American Society of Emergency Radiology)

ISMRM (International Society of Magnetic Resonance in Medicine) Meeting

ACRO (American College of Radiation Oncology) Meeting

SGR (Society of Gastrointestinal Radiologists)

May

ARRS (American Roentgen Ray Society) Meeting

ARS (American Radium Society) Meeting

SPR (Society for Pediatric Radiology) Meeting

ASNR (American Society of Neuroradiology) Meeting

APDR (Association of Program Directors in Radiology)

IPR (International Pediatric Radiology)

ISMRM (International Society for Magnetic Resonance in Medicine)

June

Oral ABR Exam (fourth year)

USMLE Exam

AMA (American Medical Association) Interim Meeting

SCAR (Society for Computer Applications in Radiology) Meeting

ASRT (American Society of Radiologic Technologists) Meeting

CAR (Canadian Association of Radiologists) Meeting

SNM (Society of Nuclear Medicine) Meeting

SUR (Society of Uroradiology) Meeting

CMRS (Clinical Magnetic Resonance Society) Meeting

ACGME (Accreditation Council for Graduate Medical Education) Meeting

July

AERS (Association of Educators in Radiological Sciences) Meeting

August

SCBT/MR (Society of Computed Body Tomography and Magnetic Resonance) Meeting

September

ACR Annual Meeting

Written ABR Exam (second, third, or fourth year)

Application deadline, ABR Exam (for following year)

Application deadline, USMLE Exam (December)

SCARD (Society of Chairmen of Academic Radiology Departments) Meeting

ICR (International Congress of Radiology)

ISS (International Skeletal Society)

ACGME (Accreditation Council for Graduate Medical Education) Meeting

October

ARRO (Association of Residents in Radiation Oncology) Meeting

SRU (Society of Radiologists in Ultrasound) Meeting

ASTRO (American Society for Therapeutic Radiology and Oncology)

RRC (Residency Review Committee) Meeting, Diagnostic Radiology

November

RSNA (Radiological Society of North America) Meeting

December

AMA (American Medical Association) Annual Meeting

Other Events (Variable Times)

AFIP Course (typically during the second or third year)

ACR State Chapter Meetings

Other Subspecialty Society Meetings

Board Review Courses

8 INSERVICE EXAM

The Annual In-Training Examination for Diagnostic Radiology Residents is sponsored by the ACR Committee on Residency Training and the Commission on Education. The purpose of the examination is to provide residents with information that are useful in evaluating their progress, and to provide program directors with data that are helpful in analyzing and evaluating their programs. The examination is intended to be a measure of general achievement in diagnostic radiology for residents and program directors and is not to be used to the detriment of a resident. All scores are strictly confidential and are reported only to Program Directors. Each Program Director should then report scores promptly to each resident. Resident scores should only be discussed between the resident and the Program Director and should not be used in any departmental discussion.

The exam contains basic science and clinical questions and lasts 3½ hours. Subsections of the exam include Musculoskeletal Radiology, Gastrointestinal Radiology, Genitourinary Radiology, Interventional Radiology, Neuroradiology, Nuclear Medicine, Pediatric Radiology, Ultrasound, Physics, Thoracic Radiology, and Mammography. The examination is open to all residents at all levels of training.

Before taking the exam, each resident must sign a consent form permitting the Program Director to have knowledge of his or her scores. The results of the individual resident scores, as well as each program's overall scores are only made available to the Program Director. Four years from the date of an individual's entry into the in-training program, all records of his or her scores are destroyed at the ACR.

9 Resident Employment and Contract Information

These sections contain multiple examples of documents relating to resident acceptance, resident contracts, and resident responsibilities. These prototypes have been adopted by the Accreditation Council for Graduate Medical Education (ACGME) and have been providing a template function since 1996. These documents were written based on the Essentials of Accredited Residencies and the Johns Hopkins Model for resident contract organization.

It should be noted that the sample departmental acceptance letter is presented in addition to the appointment letters that are sent by the hospital/school of medicine prior to the resident's acceptance of the terms listed in the resident contract.

The contract is obviously meant to be used as an outline and includes blanks and bracketed words/phrases that can be altered to meet the needs of the particular institution using the model contract. The remainder of the associated documents can be applied or not according to the needs of the particular institution or program.

All the enclosed documentation has been reviewed by various legal departments and follows the general outline for content as was originally defined by the ACGME.

These examples are presented to facilitate written agreements between residents and their institution. Preemployment expectations are also outlined to a certain degree, and many items of common concern to residents are included in the resident contract itself. Authoring these documents was a difficult but rewarding task that will hopefully provide adequate contract protection to a resident who otherwise would be at the mercy of his or her employer. All residents have the opportunity to present these contract provisions to their institution as is appropriate and can use these templates to the extent necessary to establish an equitable agreement.

1 SAMPLE DEPARTMENTAL ACCEPTANCE LETTER

Date _____

Dear _____:

On behalf of the [name of hospital] and [name of university or other associated affiliation], I am pleased to offer you a position as a house officer and position in the Department of _____ for the year beginning July___, 200___. This is a _____ year program leading to certification of residency training in _____, and is subject to annual reappointment based on satisfactory completion of the training program requirements. Participation in the program is contingent upon obtaining and maintaining a clinical appointment with [Name of hospital].

The following documents are attached and contain important information about the School of Medicine and Hospital policies. I encourage you to familiarize yourself with this information.

> Statement of responsibilities
> Financial support and benefits
> Extracurricular employment
> Procedures for discipline and redress of grievances
> Policies and procedures on sexual harassment
> Nondiscrimination policy
> Training Program Curriculum/Rotation Schedule
> Registration/Licensure.

As a member of the house staff, you will be expected to perform satisfactorily all requirements of the residency training program as described in Attachment _____. The award of a certificate of satisfactory completion of the program is conditional upon meeting all program requirements at the time of award.

You will also be expected to follow Hospital and School of Medicine policies and procedures. The University and Hospital reserve the right to modify these policies.

We look forward to your joining us and ask that you acknowledge you acceptance of this offer by signing below and returning the original copy of this letter to me.

Sincerely,

Director, _____ Residency Training Program

_____
              Signature

Attachments

2 SAMPLE STATEMENT OF RESPONSIBILITIES

The goal of the residency program is to provide trainees with an extensive training experience in the art and science of medicine in order to achieve excellence in the diagnosis, care, and treatment of patients. To achieve this goal, the trainee agrees to:

1. Under supervision of the chief of service, assume responsibilities for the safe, effective, and compassionate care of patients on the inpatient service, in the outpatient facilities, and in out-of-hospital medical care activities administered by the Hospital, consistent with the trainee's level of training and experience.

2. Participate fully in the educational and scholarly activities of the training program and, as required, assume responsibility for teaching and supervising other residency trainees and medical students.

3. Develop and participate in a personal program of self-study and professional growth with guidance from the chief of service and the teaching staff.

4. Participate in institutional programs and activities involving the medical staff and adhere to established policies, procedures, and practices of the _____ Hospital and its affiliated institutions, as assigned by the training program director.

5. Participate in institutional committees and councils, especially those that relate to patient care review activities, as determined by the program director.

6. Participate in the evaluation of education provided by the program and its teaching staff.

7. Develop an understanding of ethical, socioeconomic, and medical/legal issues that affect graduate medical education.

8. Apply cost containment measures in the provision of patient care.

3 SAMPLE RESIDENT CONTRACT

Institution Name

This agreement between [Name of hospital and appropriate affiliation] and _____ M.D./D.O. (Houseofficer) is entered into for 1 year beginning _____ and ending _____.

This agreement serves as a single statement of understanding between the Houseofficer and [Name of hospital/organization]. The term *Affiliated Hospitals,* as used herein, refers to a hospital that provides medical services to members of the public in the course of an approved medical or other professional health care clinical training program and that has an affiliation agreement with the [Name of hospital/organization] to provide that training. The term *Hospital* as used herein, refers to the specific affiliated hospital where the Houseofficer is on rotation at a given time. Each hospital is a separate entity and cannot bind any of the others through its actions.

The [Name of hospital/organization] agrees and the Houseofficer accepts appointment as a trainee under the following terms and conditions:

1. Training Program _____

2. Training Level in Program _____

3. Stipend: Level[1] _____

3. Stipend Amount $_____ per annum[2]

4. The [Name of hospital/organization] will monitor the provision of each of the following by the hospital where the Houseofficer is receiving training:

   a. Living Quarters: The Hospital shall provide suitable on-call quarters.

   b. Liability Insurance: The Hospital will provide insurance or other indemnity for liability of the Houseofficer and the Hospital while acting in the performance of his or her duties or in the course and scope of his or her assignment. Claims made after termination of training will be covered if based on acts or omissions of the Houseofficer within the course and scope of his or her assignments during training. Insurance or other liability coverage will be provided the Houseofficer on rotations outside an affiliated hospital, provided such rotation has been duly approved in writing. It is understood that a Houseofficer who participates in a rotation outside of the bounds of the Hospital and the Affiliated Hospitals is not covered by liability insurance or other indemnity.

   c. Uniforms: _____ sets of uniforms are issued [on loan/permanently] to Houseofficers. Laundering of uniforms issued to a Houseofficer will be done at no cost.

   d. Meals will be provided to an on-call Houseofficer required to spend the night in any affiliated hospital as part of his or her training program.

   e. A suitable environment will be provided for educational experience and training in the special areas of the above-named training program.

   f. Resident duty hours and on-call schedules that are not excessive.

   i. Compliance with OHSA and CDC recommendations, which assume that every direct contact with a patient's blood and other body substances is infectious and requires the use of protective equipment to prevent parenteral, mucous membrane, and nonintact skin exposures to the health care provider. The hospital agrees to provide, and make readily available, quality personal protective equipment to include gloves, face protection (masks and goggles), and cover gowns.

5. The [School of medicine/hospital], through its central payroll function, will see that the following are provided to each houseofficer:

   a. Health Insurance[3]: The Houseofficer and members of his or her immediate family, i.e., spouse and children, are eligible for enrollment in either the _____ plan or the _____ plan. If care is provided to the Houseofficer and members of his or her immediate family at one of the Affiliated Hospitals, that hospital will write off the balance of a covered procedure not paid by insurance provided under the _____ plan, after the deductible is met. Charges for services not covered under the _____ plan are the responsibility of the Houseofficer.

---

[1] May differ from level of program if credit has been given for previous training.

[2] This reflects the annual stipend for a 52-week period. Level 1 Houseofficers receive slightly more than shown [if/as] they begin a week before residents. They will be paid for 53 weeks and receive _____ of those weeks off as vacation with pay.

[3] Premium costs for these benefits are shared by the Hospital and Houseofficer for those on the [Name of hospital/organization] payroll. Houseofficers on other funding sources (stipends, fellowships, traineeships, and so forth) pay the full cost

b. Disability Insurance: A Houseofficer is eligible to participate in the [Name of hospital/organization's disability insurance plan].

c. Accident Insurance[3]: A Houseofficer is eligible to participate in [Name of hospital/organization's accident insurance plan].

d. Life Insurance[3]: A Houseofficer is eligible to participate in [Name of hospital/organization's life insurance plan].

e. Dental Insurance[3]: A Houseofficer is eligible to participate in the [Name of hospital/organization's dental insurance plan].

f. Certificate: An appropriate certificate will be provided upon satisfactory completion of the education and training program.

g. Paid Leave: Houseofficers shall receive _____ weeks off paid annual vacation if educational requirements so allow, as determined by the Program Director. Leave (to include sick, maternity/paternity, or family leave) may be taken according to written departmental policy. Leave for meetings may also be taken according to departmental policy.

6. The Houseofficer agrees to:

a. Perform satisfactorily and to the best of his or her ability the customary duties and obligations of the above-named training program as established by the training program's standards of performance.

b. Abide by the Hospital policies and procedures and the Hospital's Medical Staff bylaws, rules, and regulations.

c. Refrain from accepting fees from any patient for services rendered at the Hospital.

d. Comply with the [Name of hospital/organization] policy regarding BLS and ACLS certification for housestaff.

e. Comply with the [Name of hospital/organization] credentials verification procedure. No resident will be able to begin a training program or receive any other benefits under this agreement without having met these requirements:

  i. Provide documentation of identity and right to work.

  ii. Comply with immunization policy.

  iii. Complete the [Name of hospital/organization] application for the appointment to the housestaff, listing all information requested and returning the document in a timely manner prior to the hiring date so all information can be verified including medical school and previous residency training prior to beginning patient care responsibilities.

  iv. Obtain and maintain a valid medical license and DEA number if so required by state law.

7. The term of this agreement is for 1 year only as specifically established above, and it does not establish any right or expectation to an appointment for any subsequent residency year regardless of the number of years generally associated with a particular residency program. No agreements or representations to the contrary are valid unless introduced in writing and incorporated as a specific amendment to this agreement.

8. Due Process: Any houseofficer, hospital, or program director who disputes any action of any party shall have the right to appeal said action through the [Name of hospital/organization] due process policies, as from time to time amended. Violations of the houseofficer agreement may also be appealed in the same manner. Each houseofficer will receive a copy of said policies at the time training begins and also at the time any changes or amendments are made.

IN WITNESS WHEREOF, the parties have hereunto set their hand on the dates as hereinafter set forth.

_____   Date: _____
Houseofficer

_____   Date: _____
Training Program Director

_____   Date: _____
Director, Graduate Medical Education
[Name of hospital/organization]

4 GUIDELINES FOR RESIDENT AGREEMENT OR CONTRACTS

These guidelines replace those adopted by the American Medical Association (AMA) House of Delegates in 1974 (Report H; I-74). The earlier guidelines required revision because of changes in graduate medical education that have occurred since 1974.

The guidelines that follow are intentionally brief. They are intended to serve both residents and residency programs.

ACGME Institutional Requirements provide that residents must be provided a written agreement or contract outlining the terms and conditions of their appointment to residency training.

The AMA believes that this contract should contain or reference at least the following:

1. The resident's responsibilities, including charts, records, and reports, and the obtaining of a state licensure or educational permit, if required.
2. Financial support and benefits, including details of liability insurance,
3. Duration of appointment, conditions for reappointment, and conditions for termination,
4. Information on leave (with or without pay) that complies with federal and state laws,
5. Methods of performance evaluation
6. Policies and procedures for discipline and redress of grievances, including sexual harassment
7. Resident off-duty activities.

General Principles

The agreement or contract can take several forms. In some instances, the contract may be a detailed instrument that includes all the rules that apply to a resident's work and study and the residency program. A document can take this form when it is the outcome of negotiations between a residency organization and the institution sponsoring the residency program. The contract can, in fact, be between the institution and a resident organization instead of individual residents.

The document frequently takes the form of a relatively brief contract or a letter of agreement setting forth matters that apply to individual residents and referring to other documents—such as a resident handbook or set of hospital rules—that explain all the rules residents are expected to observe.

Both a contract and a letter of agreement are binding on both parties. Whatever form the document takes, it should, to the extent possible, be the same for all residents and fellows in an institution. (For convenience, the document and referenced material will be referred to as a "contract" hereafter.)

The obligations of both parties to the agreement should be stated, either in the contract, or in the referenced material. In general, the institution agrees to provide an educational program for the resident that, at a minimum, meets the standards established by the ACGME during the term of the contract and also to provide salary and benefits. The resident agrees to meet the educational requirements of the program and to provide safe, effective, and compassionate care under the supervision of residency faculty. The resident is also obligated to comply with state and federal laws and regulations as well as established policies.

ACGME Requirements

ACGME accreditation requirements are binding on both the institution and the resident. The ACGME requirements may be referenced in the contract. ACGME requirements provide for work hours and supervision regulations, as well as rules concerning the content of education and the amount of required exposure to certain procedures. The ACGME requirements are not subject to negotiation.

Salaries

The contract should specify the amount of salary to be paid to a resident and the intervals at which payment will be made. Either the contract or the referenced material should indicate when salary increments will be made and the basis for such increments. Although residents at the same level in different programs in the institution should, to the extent possible, be paid the same salary, a differential may be paid for senior residents. (Note: court decisions may in the near future establish that ACGME cannot require that all residents at the same level be paid the same amount.)

Work Hours

Work hours expected of the resident should be specified in the contract. Basic principals concerning work hours are provided in ACGME Institutional Requirements. Exact limitations on work hours are stated in the ACGME Program Requirements for each specialty field. Work hours requirements must not exceed ACGME limits. In general, residents should have one full day out of seven free of program duties, and, on average, on call duties no more than every third night.

Leave

The amount of vacation, sick leave, and educational leave should be specified, as should any limitations as to the times of year when vacation can be taken. Information must be provided as to family leave, bereavement leave, and education leave. The contract should state whether expenses are provided for attending medical conferences.

Insurance Benefits

The contract should provide detailed information about insurance benefits, including the kinds of insurance provided (e.g., life insurance, health insurance, and disability insurance), whether premiums are paid by the program or the resident, who is covered by the policies (i.e., the resident and spouse and children), and what is covered. The contract must also provide information concerning the professional liability insurance provided, including "tail" provisions. In general, residents should be provided with insurance benefits commensurate with those provided to other staff in the institution. If it is the practice to provide medical care for the resident instead of insurance, the contract should indicate the kinds and amounts of medical care that can be provided.

Off-Duty Activities and Employment

In general, a resident's time after the completion of duties is not subject to the program's control. The program can require that residents be rested and alert while performing their duties. The program director is responsible for addressing a resident's fitness for performance of duties.

Sexual Harassment and Antidiscrimination Policies

The contract should include or make reference to the policy concerning sexual harassment, as well the policy concerning equal employment opportunity.

Terms and Condition of Appointment and Reappointment

The contract should set out the duration of the appointment and the conditions for reappointment.

Termination of Appointment

The contract should provide the circumstances in which a residency appointment can be terminated and the procedures to be followed in such a termination. These procedures should provide the resident an opportunity to rebut the allegations given for termination and should provide the opportunity for counsel.

Grievance Procedures

The contract should include grievance procedures or reference published grievance procedures. These procedures should include a definition of grievance, a statement as to the right of an individual resident to initiate a grievance procedure, a description of the procedures, including an indication of how the procedures will be concluded, and the right of the resident to counsel.

Disciplinary Procedures

The contract should indicate the circumstances and procedures for disciplinary hearings and the disciplinary actions that can be taken.

Closing of Facilities or Residency Programs

The contract must include provision for residents in case of such closure. Residents should receive treatment equal to that provided other staff affected by the closing. This should include notification of a projected closing as early as possible, as well as payment of salary and benefits to the conclusion of the contract. Provisions should also be made for the proper disposition of residency education records, including appropriate notification to licensure and specialty boards.

Ancillary Support

The contract should include information regarding living quarters, meals, laundry, or their equivalents.

5 CURRICULUM VITAE PREPARATION, LOCUMS TENENS, AND MOONLIGHTING

Curriculum Vitae

The origin of the term is Latin and means *the course of one's life or career.* Your CV is a word picture of yourself. You must communicate a clear impression about yourself, your background, and your qualifications. Put together an organized, attractive, and concise document that makes note of your accomplishments. It has to be clear and understandable the first time through. Although there is not an optimal length, it is best to be concise. There are verbose two-page CVs and concise five-page summaries. Unless you are widely published, or have years of experiences, attempt to stay within two to three pages. This will prevent the reader from losing interest. Check and double-check the document for misspellings and poor grammar (grammar and spelling must be perfect). Revise and perfect your CV over the course of time by taking the best style elements from various CVs you happen to encounter.

There are many styles and formats for a CV. One style is as follows:

1. Name
2. Address and telephone number
3. Career objectives
4. Education:
   a. College
   b. Graduate school
   c. Medical school
5. Board certification
6. Medical licensure
7. Professional memberships and societies
8. Honors and awards
9. Work experience (candidates with more extensive clinical job experience will probably want to list their job experience before the education category), in chronologic order:
   a. Jobs held for a significant time
   b. Jobs applicable to medicine
   c. Military experience
10. Research positions/experience/interests
11. Publications/bibliography

12. Presentations
13. Special training, languages
14. Personal data (optional):
    a. Marital status
    b. Children
    c. Citizenship
15. References (optional).

Locums Tenens/Moonlighting

Moonlighting offers residents an opportunity to broaden their clinical experience, learn about communities in which they might want to practice, let the practice learn more about them, and find out what clinical practice is like outside a tertiary care center. Most importantly, it lets you experience what it is like to take on a professional's responsibilities.

Most residency programs have rules about moonlighting. Some allow more extensive moonlighting, and others don't allow any. Most restrict moonlighting to either specific amounts of time or situations in which it will not interfere with resident activities. States may also regulate moonlighting through licen-

sure. A number of states require 2 or more years of postgraduate training prior to licensure. If you think you might want to moonlight, find out under what conditions it is allowed in your program and state.

The next question is whether moonlighting jobs are available. In some institutions, moonlighting opportunities exist within the institution itself or at the institution's satellite facilities. In other programs, groups of residents have established relationships with local practices where moonlighting opportunities are available. In most cases, however, finding moonlighting opportunities is an individual endeavor. Try to find out whether current residents have found such opportunities. Liability insurance is an absolute must for all residents moonlighting. If there are moonlighting opportunities within the institution, the cost of the liability insurance may not be covered by your institution. In other cases, the radiology practice you are moonlighting for will furnish insurance. If you are forced to get your own insurance, it can be very expensive. Talk to the current residents to find out about moonlighting and liability insurance in your area.

6 FINDING A JOB

Services of the ACR Professional Bureau Available to Residents and Fellows

The Professional Bureau of the American College of Radiology (ACR) is a source of job opening information and contacts for ACR members who are either seeking a new position or seeking an individual to fill a position. This is a free service to ACR members. Residents and fellows are given a temporary complementary membership and are encouraged to use these services. *In the fall, letters are sent to fourth-year residents and to fellows in the last year of their fellowship training inviting them to use the ACR Professional Bureau Service to aid them in their search for a position.*

THE ON-LINE SERVICE

The ACR Professional Bureau is on the internet and can be accessed whether you are registered with the Bureau or not. The internet listings are updated every Saturday. The web address is http://www.acr.org, and a user name and password are needed to access these listings.

Access Information

ACR member passwords used in other protected areas of the College's Website do not work in the Professional Bureau area. Access is restricted to those with an active listing and/or to ACR members who have registered to browse the listing. Once registered, you will need to choose a password to access the listings. This will be good for as long as your listing is active. If you allow your listing or registration to expire, you will need to submit a new form, wait for it to be activated, and then select a new password. New participants will not be able to search the

listings until their individual listing is activated. This usually takes 1 or 2 business days after the submission of the Listing Form or Browser Registration.

For ACR members, your user name is the first letter of your first name and the first letter of your last name in capital letters, followed by your member number with no spaces or punctuation. For example, Jane Williams would be JW plus your ACR member number (JW1234567). After entering that, hit the TAB key and enter your password, which is your ACR member number by itself (based on the above example: 1234567). Members of the American Society for Therapeutic Radiology and Oncology (ASTRO) and nonmembers with paid listings should contact the Professional Bureau for their user name after they submit the listing form. If you need help in determining your ACR membership number, call the ACR Professional Bureau at 1-800-227-3370.

Professional Bureau applicants must be available for employment within 12 months of their listing date. (Candidates for fellowship openings may list up to 18 months prior to availability.) Your information will appear in the web listings and in the monthly paper bulletin sent to those participants listing with the bureau who do not have web access. Each listing is active for 6 months and may be renewed in 6-month increments. To be listed, you need to register with the ACR Professional Bureau.

INTERVIEWS AT MEETINGS

The ACR Professional Bureau also offers on-site interview services at meetings such as those of ASTRO in the fall and of the Radiological Society of North America (RSNA) in December. These interview services offer the opportunity for applicants and employers to meet each other face to face. Both employers and applicants may preregister to participate in meeting interviews, or they may register on site. Applicants must meet the availability criteria mentioned above. Watch the web site for announcements of interview services at future meetings.

SUMMARY POINTS

– Residents and fellows may visit the ACR Professional Bureau's internet site at any time.

– You may register to be listed with the ACR Professional Bureau only 12 months prior to your availability for employment and 18 months prior to your availability for a fellowship position.

– Call the ACR Professional Bureau at 1-800-227-3370 if you have any additional questions.

Getting A Job

Getting a job is one of the biggest concerns of radiology residents across the country. Indeed, this is one of the biggest subjects in the minds of all radiology residents. It should be noted, however, that radiology has one of the lowest unemployment rates among the various specialties. Residents are concerned about finding jobs, but almost all eventually find one (according to ACR research). Although this is true, it does not diminish the stress and anxiety experienced by fourth-year residents and fellows. This section will review the process of job hunting and provide tips to make the process a little easier.

The process of getting a job begins early in residency. The first question to be answered is what route to take, academic or private practice. Residents should reflect upon their own interests and career goals. There is no right or wrong answer, and individuals need to determine their own personal preferences. Participating in research and preparing lectures are ways that one can try the academic way of life. Additionally, discussions with academic faculty and members of local private practices are good sources of information. Preparations for either career should optimally begin early, but it is not rare to find residents who have not committed to a definite career track at the time of graduation.

If an academic career is contemplated, academic endeavors such as publication, exhibits, scientific presentations, and lectures will help build the appropriate CV. Promotion and tenure in the academic arena is largely based on accomplishments listed in the CV. This type of work relatively early in residency will help you get an academic job and provide a springboard for later promotions and tenure after the job is secured. At least trying one or two projects is useful, even if you are certain you will be going into private practice. Although it is not absolutely necessary to do research in residency to get an academic job, the academic experience does make you a stronger candidate.

Contacts are very helpful in the job market. If you have a strong desire to practice in a specific locale, get to know the practicing radiologists in this area. When groups hire a new person, they would rather hire someone they know and like. It is not difficult to make contacts with radiologists in the locale of your residency. For example, most residency programs are within the geographic domain of a radiology society. The society may encompass all the radiologists of a city or a region of the state. If the society has meetings or other functions and you would like to make your home in that area, consider going to the society's events. This form of networking is extremely important.

That seems to be easy enough, but what if you want to practice in an area that is not in the vicinity of your residency program? One option is to look for moonlighting opportunities in that area. This is a great opportunity for the radiologists of a given practice to see how you perform "in the trenches." Even if you are moonlighting at night or on the weekend, the members of the practice usually seek feedback from technologists and clinicians about you. If your work ethic was lacking or you did not interact well with the clinical and technologic staff, it may be difficult to compete for any future positions in the group. However, you will make a more favorable impression if you do your work well, efficiently, and as a team member.

If no moonlighting opportunities are available, you may want to write a letter to a few select groups in the region outlining your interests. A meeting or telephone call would be useful to make a contact or two. This initial contact is useful in the early to mid-stages of your residency. A good approach toward arranging this initial contact is to solicit advice regarding your goal of eventually practicing in that area. This is a direct and honest approach that clearly declares your career goals to the practice members. Additional contacts over the subsequent time in residency can help to foster your relationships with these radiologists. This familiarity cannot be overemphasized. It is human nature to hire someone that you know and like.

In the past, many residents graduated from residency programs and immediately went into a practice. Some residents still take this direct approach. Many residents, however, are presently doing fellowships. The fellowship makes you more attractive in a competitive market. You will potentially bring more subspecialty expertise and more experience to potential employers. The market demands may also significantly increase the importance of doing fellowships. In some regions, nearly all the graduating residents do a fellowship. Hence, a fellowship can be critical to getting a good job in popular areas of the country.

Regardless of whether or not you do a fellowship, the most important determinant of your job competitiveness is your ability to do radiology. Employers want trustworthy, pleasant individuals who are able to do high-quality radiology. They do not want individuals who are not comfortable with many modalities or procedures, must be supervised on a regular basis, cannot be counted on to do their share of the work, or, most importantly, are not competent for patient care. Along with the present changes in health care, there is a greater emphasis on accountability and quality assurance. Practice groups cannot afford to lower their credibility in the realm of patient care. Certification through the American Board of Radiology (ABR) is a very important support for your competence as a radiologist. Managed care organizations and hospital credentialing may place a great deal of importance on ABR certification. All you can do is work hard during residency and learn as much as you can. Do not assume you will become a good radiologist, rather, work hard to make yourself an excellent radiologist.

When it does come time to apply for jobs, there are several things to keep in mind. The ACR Professional Bureau is a very good resource for job searching. The active listings are excellent to review and for initial inquiries. You can quickly evaluate and focus on job listings that are the most relevant and attractive for your career interests. Additionally, you can list yourself through the placement bureau as someone looking for a job. However, if it is a buyers market, you will need to write more letters and make more phone calls than you will receive. Send your CV to many groups and follow the letters up with telephone calls.

As stated previously, networking is also a very important way to look for good jobs. Talk to faculty, your mentor, and local contacts about jobs they have heard about. Not infrequently, one or more of these people will have a friend that is looking to hire. You may learn of jobs that you would not have otherwise. Additionally, the person advising you about the job

may be a good reference to help you find a job. Again, people like to hire candidates they know and candidates who are recommended by a friend.

Try not to be too restrictive in the type of job you apply for and the geographic region. The more limitations you make, the more difficult it will be to secure a good job. Be willing to check into jobs that initially may not appear attractive, as you may be pleasantly surprised. Certain geographic locations may have an unpopular reputation but may actually be good places to live. The nature of the job can also be misleading. Certain job listings may not seem attractive on the surface but may have more promise when you gain more details. Unfortunately, the reverse is probably a more frequent occurrence. Job listings are made to appear attractive but may have undesirable features under the surface. The bottom line is to keep an open mind but stay cautious.

It is also important not to be too restrictive in the particular modalities you are willing to work. Do not assume that you will be working in a certain subspecialty just because you are fellowship trained in that area. The service demands of a practice have to be met and require a certain flexibility of practice members to work in other areas/modalities of radiology.

7 YOUR PROFESSIONAL CONTRACT: *WHAT YOU SHOULD KNOW*

Introduction: *The Professional Contract*

An employment contract is probably the most important document that a young physician encounters in his or her early professional life, a document that turns an offer of employment into a defined employment relationship. Contracts typically involve hundreds of thousands of dollars in salary and other benefits, as well as binding commitments that may severely limit an individual's professional opportunities. It is also a document that most physicians are ill prepared to assess, given the lack of emphasis on business and legal issues in traditional education. This makes it all the more important to seek competent legal advice regarding the specific terms of a contract and hopefully learn to recognize its key features.

Features of a Typical Contract

An employment contract usually includes several basic provisions, such as terms of employment, salary, and benefits, although not always in predictable order. In addition to these basic provisions, many contracts will often contain numerous other clauses that supply the finer details of the employment relationship. Typical features include:

1. *Terms of employment.* A contract will typically recite the type of practice you are entering, i.e., proprietorship, partnership, professional corporation, and so forth, and your relationship to that entity, i.e., an employee, a partner, shareholder, or other. Your duties to the practice will usually be outlined. Outside medical employment is ordinarily prohibited; income from

other sources, such as book revenues, speaking fees, and consulting fees may or may not become the property of your group. It is important to examine this section closely, as its terms will often vary with the practice setting and geographic location.

2. *Salary.* The amount of compensation and when that compensation comes due for all years covered by the contract should be included. If a bonus is involved, it is desirable to have the terms of that compensation spell out, i.e., when it will be paid, how it will be computed, and so forth.

3. *Opportunity for partnership.* Shares in the corporation or similar ownership status. If consideration for partnership, shareholder status, and so on is anticipated, the time at which you will be evaluated for this status should be stated. If the practice has a buy-in requirement, the terms of that buy-in should be prospectively defined. A buy-out provision, allowing you to recover your investment if you leave, should always be included in the presence of a substantial buy-in.

4. *Malpractice insurance and related expenses.* Important provisions include who will pay for this insurance, what the coverage entails, and who assumes the cost of a "tail" for claims made on policies.

5. *Practice expenses and support staff.* Costs associated with your practice, such as home-based teleradiology equipment, office expenses, and so on, if reimbursed by the practice, should be included in the contract. Ideally, provisions for support staff you feel necessary, such as nurses, technologists, or secretaries, should be part of the document.

6. *Benefits.* Health, life, and disability coverage, if employer provided, should be described in the contract. Also important are

retirement plans, which can constitute a large portion of the compensation package.

7. *Vacation time, sick leave, call schedule, and meeting time.* All should be defined in the contract. For new physicians in a group, it is not uncommon for vacation time, sick leave, on-call time, or meeting time to be expressed in terms of what partners or other senior members of the practice are receiving. A dollar amount available for meeting expenses is also desirable.

8. *Incidental expenses.* Groups will often cover moving expenses, license fees, and membership in professional organizations; occasionally, club memberships will also be included. It is always desirable to have these benefits recited in the contract.

9. *Termination of employment.* Most contracts allow for termination with advance notice by either party and also for automatic termination under certain circumstances, such as loss of medical license or hospital privileges. Be aware that some contracts may limit your right to leave the group during the contract period.

10. *Covenant not to compete.* Nearly all contracts include clauses that limit your ability to practice in a varying area around your employer's facilities for some length of time following the termination of your employment. These clauses also severely limit your access to the group's records and patients should you leave. If the terms of these provisions are reasonable, they are usually legally enforceable. This is particularly true if there is a "liquidated damages" section, which assigns a certain dollar amount of damages should you break the covenant.

Observation and Recommendations

Employment contracts are very variable legal documents and differ widely in their provisions and details. There is no such thing as a perfect contract. From a legal perspective, it is better to have more detail rather than less, particularly where there may be a point of contention. Practically, an employer may be quite reluctant to change some or all of his or her contract's provisions, and even the most amicable employer usually tolerates only a round or two of contract revisions. As difficult as it may be to raise potentially contentious issues with a prospective employer, failure to settle significant differences in the contract negotiation process may lead to serious disputes in the course of employment.

It is strongly recommended that a physician seek competent legal advice before signing any employment contract. The attorney reviewing the document should be knowledgeable regarding the legal aspects of radiology employment in the geographic location of the employment opportunity. Such caution, although sometimes initially expensive, may prevent a substantially more costly mistake.

8 MISCELLANEOUS ADVICE FOR FINDING AND SECURING A JOB

Potential Pitfalls

GETTING A JOB

Obtain or review the ACR's job listings early in residency and look for openings that repeat every so often through the years, especially in seemingly desirable locations to practice. This may be evidence of "churning" of physician employees by the practice, i.e., hiring someone out of residency or fellowship with the promise of future partnership in the practice but "letting the hiree go" sometime short of partnership and then hiring a new candidate to fill the position. This is an unfortunate reality of today's hiring practice by many radiology groups.

There is no such thing as a "perfect job." When looking for a job, a good exercise to do is to list your priorities (geographic location, group size, term to partnership, and so on) and then attempt to find a position that has the best combination of your listed priorities. A typical tradeoff under this scenario would be taking a position in a less desirable geographic location in exchange for a more secure job position.

YOUR PROFESSIONAL CONTRACT

Insist on a signed contract with all the details worked out prior to starting a new job. "We will work out the details when you get here" or "you'll get your formal contract once you start work" are hollow promises and could lead to significant employment problems regarding what was promised and what eventually gets delivered to the employed physician.

Have your potential contract reviewed by an attorney from the state where the job position is located. There may be significant differences in state statutes regarding employment and employees rights.

FEATURES OF A TYPICAL CONTRACT

Look out for the ploy of buying into the group's accounts receivable as part of the buy-in. Typically, you have already "earned" these receivables by accepting to work at a lower salary than the partners in the radiology group. You would end up paying twice for those receivables.

Get everything you feel is important in writing in the contract. People have short memories when it comes to verbal agreements. Also, don't ask for unreasonable terms in the contract; this may not win you favor with the other radiologists in the group, especially if what you are asking for is something they do not have.

A good source of information on the business of medicine, including contracts, is *Medical Economics* magazine. Read exerpts from this periodical if you have the time. You can learn a substantial amount about many different subjects that may not seem important during training or in the first few years of practice, but will be in the future (i.e., pension plans, estate planning, employment contract, and so on).

9 TRANSITION TO RADIOLOGY PRACTICE

Congratulations! You're back from Louisville and most likely have passed the ABR Oral Examination that has been the primary focus of your attention for the past few months. Five long years of studying, short nights, and long days have culminated in a successful trip to the Executive West, and you have just received or will soon receive the letter confirming your success in attaining board certification.

After the intensity of the months gone by, you are looking forward to the casual four to six weeks before beginning your fellowship or before starting that job that you selected the previous fall. Having become accustomed to the frantic and anxiety-provoking past few months, it is time to break the study cycle and reintroduce yourself to your spouse/significant other and children and to see what other portions of your life have survived the pre-Boards neglect.

Despite the excitement and relief that accompanies a successful attempt at board certification, your respite will be brief. You are about to begin a complex process called Transition to Practice, during which you will go from the comfortable environment you know well to unfamiliar territory. Just as you give time and consideration to packing for a long trip or your likely upcoming move, the next few weeks are a time to gather the resources you need to make the transition as easy as possible. For your assistance, here is a list of things you will probably need and various suggestions to ease the transition from resident to fellow or attending staff.

Paperwork

Between you and the final destination of radiology practice stands a legion of people who want you to fill out forms. Although the venerable ABR has certified you as a radiologist, you must now obtain credentials from your new hospital(s), managed care insurance companies, Preferred Provider Organizations, and a variety of other organizations, including the state medical board if you are moving to a new state.

This is essentially a process of making sure you are who you say you are and have trained to the level you say you have. Fortunately, many of these people want similar information, and many of these documents should already be in your possession. Others will be provided to you during the exit process. Organization is an absolute necessity in successfully navigating this process. If you have engaged in locums tenens (moonlighting) during your residency, some of this process will be familiar and you will already have collected a number of these documents. The pile of documents is sure to grow, and developing some kind of filing system is recommended to ensure that you will preserve and be able to retrieve the necessary documents easily.

Documents that you will soon need include:

– Medical school diploma

– Board Certification Certificate

– Internship Training Certificate

– Residency Training Certificate

– Fellowship Training Certificate (if you have one)

– Drug Enforcement Agency (DEA) license

– State controlled substances permit

– Basic Life Support (BLS)/Advanced Cardiac Life Support (ACLS) Certificate (BLS is usually required/ACLS is recommended)

– Birth certificate or other citizenship/immigration papers

– State license and current permit (varies from state to state)

– Medicare UPIN number (if you have one)

– Reference letters from other physicians (usually three individuals).

If you have access to a notary at your program (you probably do; ask around) and you are staying in the same state, have notarized copies of your diploma, Board Certification, and birth certificate (or other citizenship papers) made *before* you have them framed. This way, you can produce notarized copies of these documents before becoming established at your new practice or in your new fellowship. If you are moving to a new state and require a new license, it is important to start this process as soon as possible. The medical license application process usually takes 3 to 6 months or more, and some states have specific requirements (e.g., a jurisprudence exam in Texas) that require advance preparation.

Other documentation you need will come from your program, and this will vary depending on your mode of practice and the modalities you will cover. Although mammography is the only subspecialty that requires a specific number of examinations to be interpreted prior to residency completion, the ACGME program requirements state that each resident must have documented supervised experience in various interventional procedures. These may include, but are not limited to, image-guided biopsies, drainage procedures, noncoronary angioplasty, embolization and infusion procedures, and percutaneous introduction techniques. These requirements also state that the program director must require the residents to maintain a record (electronic or written) in which they document the performance, interpretation, and complications of vascular, interventional, and invasive procedures.

Your program director or subspecialty instructors should provide you with letters detailing your level of training in:

– Mammography

– Stereotactic Breast Biopsy

– Vascular Ultrasound

– Obstetrical Ultrasound

– Interventional procedures

– Nuclear Medicine (including both diagnostic and therapeutic indications)

– Magnetic Resonance Imaging

– Conscious Sedation (if appropriate)

It is a good idea to have as many modalities documented as possible maximizing your options in light of the growing prevalence of certification in fields such as mammography, ultrasound, and magnetic resonance imaging. In addition to being useful for certification purposes, documentation of modality experience will assist your former residency program to demonstrate its compliance with modality exposure requirements. These guidelines specifically state that residents must have training and experience in plain film interpretation, computed tomography, magnetic resonance imaging, ultrasonography, angiography, and nuclear radiology examinations related to cardiovascular disease.

When possible, they should document the exact number of cases you have participated in, particularly for nuclear medicine, mammography, and stereotactic breast biopsy. These records should also document the number of months spent in each field and the approximate number of cases seen, in per unit time (i.e., per week or per month). As stated previously, you should have been documenting these numbers yourself during the course of your training, but adequately organized radiology and hospital information systems databases should also be able to produce these numbers for you quickly and accurately. It is useful for residents to persuade their programs to provide them with a list of their procedures by Current Procedural Terminology (CPT) code (minus patient identification) at various intervals throughout the residency. This will facili-

tate an accurate and up-to-date documentation method that requires little time investment by the resident.

To meet the Food and Drug Administration's Mammography Quality Standards Act requirements, a resident must have at least 3 months of training in the interpretation of mammograms including instruction in radiation physics, radiation effects, and radiation protection. These requirements also state that the resident must have read or interpreted (under the direct supervision of an interpreting physician) the mammograms from the examinations of at least 240 patients within a 6-month period. If the resident passed the certifying board examination in diagnostic radiology at the first allowable time (i.e., the earliest time a resident is eligible to take the board certification exam), the 6-month period could have been any time within the last 2 years of the residency program. If a resident conditions *any* section of the oral board examination and wishes to read mammography, the individual must read 240 mammograms in the 6 months preceding departure from residency. Therefore, as insurance against this eventuality, senior residents may want to be sure they read 240 mammograms between January 1 before the boards and the end of residency. If you have not and you condition any section of the oral board examination, you must read an additional 240 mammograms before your final day of residency. To abide by the final regulations of the Quality Standards Act, the resident must present a letter from his or her residency program director to their mammography facility. An example of such as letter is listed below:

Sample Residency Letter Final Regulations

The following letter should be on the official letterhead of the residency program:

May 25, 2001

To Whom It May Concern:

Dr. [Name of physician] successfully completed his/her residency in diagnostic radiology on [Date]. During the period of his/her residency program [List inclusive dates], Dr. [Name] received the following training and experience specific to mammography:

1. At least 3 months [This statement may or may not include the exact amount of Training] of training in the interpretation of mammograms, including instruction in radiation physics, radiation effects, and radiation protection. [*Note:* This paragraph may be deleted if the resident has passed the diagnostic radiology certifying examinations and become a diplomat of the ABR, the American Osteopathic Board of Radiology (AOBR), or the Royal College of Physicians and Surgeons of Canada (RCPSC).]

2. At least 60 hours of documented continuing medical education in mammography. [*Note to residency program director:* These 60 hours may be included in the 3 months of training described in #1; this does not have to be an additional 60 hours of training.]

3. Read or interpreted, under the direct supervision of an interpreting physician, the mammograms from the examinations of at least 240 patients within the 6-month period of [Give the dates of the 6-month period]

or

If the resident physician passed the certifying board examination in diagnostic radiology at the first allowable time, the 6-month period could have been any time within the last 2 years of the residency program [Give dates of 6-month period]. [*Note:* The "first allowable time" means the earliest time that a resident physician is eligible to take the certifying examination.]

_____

[Signed by an official of the Residency Program]

_____

[Must include signing official's title, e.g., Chairman of Program, Director of Residency Education, Director of Mammography Section]

Intellectual Property

As a radiology resident for the last 4 years, you have no doubt become comfortable with the way in which exams are performed at your hospital. Your interpretation patterns have been shaped by the protocols and methods used at your hospital, and these are a form of psychological security you can take with you to your eventual practice site. It is far easier to obtain standard forms, preprinted orders, and protocol sheets before you leave than to construct them from scratch once you realize you need them. These documents should also be stored in your organized filing system as well.

Obviously, a certain amount of tact and political finesse is required as well as the direct permission that is needed before you copy the protocols with the express intent of taking them to another institution. There will also undoubtedly be a certain set of standard protocols and a certain way business is done wherever you go (especially if you are a fellow and are supposed to be learning). Nevertheless, some degree of flexibility is accorded to new staff-level physicians, and you should exercise that enough to make yourself comfortable. Moreover, as a recently trained radiologist, you are expected to bring new techniques and improved protocols that reflect some of the advances of the modern practice of radiology and its subspecialties.

Forms to appropriate or create include things such as:

- Computed tomography protocols (slice thickness, contrast rates and timings, window/level, kVp/mAs, pitch, and so on)
- Magnetic resonance imaging protocols (type of sequence, TR, TE, FOV, matrix, NEX, bandwidth, flip angle, type of contrast, and so on.)
- Interventional protocols (contrast rates and dosages, imaging planes and rates)
- Nuclear medicine protocols
  - Dosages and agents
  - Imaging protocols (seconds for each image, window settings, and so on.)
- Preprinted orders (postcatheterization, postbiopsy, for example)
- Consent forms (for ideas; your new site probably has its own)
- Printing protocols for computed tomography and magnetic resonance imaging
- Standard negative dictations
- Report forms for specific modalities
- Staff and technologist phone list.

Most experienced magnetic resonance imaging and computed tomography technologists can take a printed study from your training site and do their best to duplicate it in terms of pulse sequence, slice thickness, and order of printing. This is particularly helpful if you are introducing an innovative technique or a modality upgrade to your new practice.

If you plan to do interventional procedures, attempt to document the manufacturer and model number of every catheter, wire, and other device for which you have affection. Nothing is worse than getting some strange device handed to you during your first procedure at a new place and trying to figure out what it is while the technologists watch you and giggle. When just beginning in a new practice, it is surprising how much confidence something as prosaic as a familiar biopsy gun or catheter will provide.

An additional and vital piece of information, particularly if you are introducing a new procedure at your practice site, is a CPT code list. *Do not* bring a list of charges to your new practice. They will set their own charges and by attempting to incorporate the charges from another practice verbatim, you could run afoul of antitrust law. The CPT code will aid your billing department in defining and appropriately charging any new procedures. This happens more commonly than you would imagine, especially if you are going to a smaller hospital than your tertiary-care training site.

General Housekeeping

Before you leave your program (and before you switch insurance), have a physical and get a letter stating the date the exam was performed and that you have no physical or mental impairments that will prevent you from practicing in a safe manner. If your residency program offers discounted prescriptions, be sure these are filled before you leave. If you have moonlighting malpractice insurance, be sure to buy out the "tail" and keep this document—your new malpractice insurance company will want it, and many hospital staff applications will have a list of malpractice insurance policies you have had in the past, including dates.

If you have had the misfortune to be involved in a malpractice case that has not closed, get the name and number of your hospital counsel and be sure they know where you are headed. For closed cases, you will probably need a brief listing of the circumstances and disposition of any cases in which you have been named. These are all going to be in the National Practitioners Data Bank report that the medical staff at your new practice site will order, and an explanation will be required. If you are under the care of a physician for any problem, have a letter available explaining your condition and its implications for your practice, if any.

If you have privileges at other hospitals for moonlighting, keep a list of the addresses of these places and the phone number of the medical staff offices. Send them a letter requesting that you be placed on inactive status. If they require you to resign, be sure they send you a letter stating that you resigned in good standing and without quality or patient relation issues, and keep this letter with you.

Contact the state medical licensing boards of all of the states where you hold licenses, informing them of your new address and practice location. Some of these boards may also offer the option of converting your license to an inactive status. The inactive status will not allow you to practice in that state but will allow you to keep your state license at a reduced annual fee. Reactivating an inactive license is much easier than reapplying for a new license, and this option should be considered if you have any inclination at all of returning to that particular state to practice or intend to read any teleradiology images from there.

If you have letters of recommendation or evaluation forms that need to be completed by staff at your training program, be sure that those individuals you asked to do you this favor actually complete the requested task. Failure to obtain letters of reference will cause undue delays in your credentialing and will also cause the medical staff in charge of the credentialing process more work, as their oversight of your credentials confirmation will be prolonged. Staying informed and current on the status of the credentialing process at your future site can prevent unnecessary delays. Also, politely asking the staff writing your letters and forms to finish them before you leave is much more effective than handling this situation after your departure.

Give your program director, department director, and educational assistant a token of your gratitude and affection. These individuals will undoubtedly have to help you in the future and have most likely provided valuable assistance in the past, so try to leave on the best terms possible.

Conclusions

Your actions taken in the final weeks of your residency can make your future life substantially less stressful, particularly if you are moving a significant distance from your training site. The lack of a piece of critical documentation means long-distance phone calls, registered mail, privilege delays, and possibly payment delays. In addition, what is now immediately vital to you is of secondary importance to people at your program because their time is currently being occupied by other concerns directly related to their present trainees. Both private practice and academic radiology can be personally and professionally rewarding; with some strategically coordinated efforts properly placed, you can quickly get down to the enjoyable business of radiology practice.

10 Resident Requirements

1. INSTITUTIONAL REQUIREMENTS

Institutional Organization and Commitment

The purpose of graduate medical education (GME) is to provide an organized educational program with guidance and supervision of the resident, facilitating the resident's professional and personal development while ensuring safe and appropriate care for patients. Sponsoring institutions, therefore, must be appropriately organized for the conduct of GME in a scholarly environment and be committed to excellence in both education and medical care. This commitment is exhibited by the provision of leadership and resources to enable the institution to achieve substantial compliance with the Institutional Requirements and to enable the educational programs to achieve substantial compliance with Program Requirements. This includes providing an ethical and professional environment in which the educational curricular requirements, as well as the applicable requirements for scholarly activity, can be met. Regular assessment of the quality of the educational programs is an essential component of this commitment.

SPONSORING INSTITUTION

1. A residency program must operate under the authority and control of a sponsoring institution.
2. There must be a written statement of institutional commitment to GME that is supported by the governing authority, the administration, and the teaching staff.
3. Sponsoring institutions must be in substantial compliance with the Institutional Requirements and must ensure that their

Accreditation Council for Graduate Medical Education (ACGME)-accredited programs are in substantial compliance with the Program Requirements.
4. An institution's failure to comply substantially with the Institutional Requirements may jeopardize the accreditation of all of its sponsored residency programs.

EDUCATIONAL ADMINISTRATION

There must be an organized administrative system to oversee all residency programs sponsored by an institution. In addition, there must be a designated institutional official who has the authority and the responsibility for the oversight and administration of the GME programs.

1. Institutions must have a GME Committee (GMEC) that has the responsibility for monitoring and advising on all aspects of residency education. Voting membership on the committee must include residents nominated by their peers, appropriate program directors, other members of the faculty, and the accountable institutional official or his or her designee.
2. The committee must meet at least quarterly; minutes must be kept and be available for inspection by accreditation personnel.
3. The responsibilities of the committee must include:
   a. Establishment and implementation of policies that affect all residency programs regarding the quality of education and the work environment for the residents in each program.
   b. Establishment and maintenance of appropriate oversight of and liaison with program directors and assurance that

Source: Accreditation Council for Graduate Medical Education (ACGME), September , 1998; effective, September, 1998. *Graduate Medical Education Directory, 2001–2002,* American Medical Association.

program directors establish and maintain proper oversight of and liaison with appropriate personnel of other institutions participating in programs sponsored by the institutions.

c. Regular review of all residency programs to assess their compliance with both the Institutional Requirements and Program Requirements of the relevant ACGME Residency Review Committees (RRCs).

i The review must be conducted by the GMEC or a body designated by the GMEC, which should include faculty, residents, and administrators, both within and outside the department in which the residency exists. The review must follow a written protocol approved by the GMEC. External reviewers may also be utilized as determined by the GMEC.

ii. Reviews must be conducted between the ACGME program surveys.

Iii While assessing the residency program's compliance with each of the program standards, the review should also appraise the following:

(a) The educational objectives of each program

(b) The adequacy of available educational and financial resources to meet these objectives

(c) The effectiveness of each program in meeting its objectives

(d) The effectiveness in addressing citations from previous ACGME letters of accreditation and previous internal reviews.

iv. Examples of materials and data to be used in the review process should include the following:

(a) Institutional and Program Requirements from the Essentials of Accredited Residency Programs

(b) Letters of accreditation from previous ACGME reviews

(c) Reports from previous internal reviews of the program

(d) Interviews with the program director, faculty, and residents in the program and individuals outside the program deemed appropriate by the committee.

v. There must be documentation of the review, including recorded mechanisms to correct identified deficiencies. In addition, succinct summaries of each review are required as part of the ACGME institutional review document.

vi. Although departmental annual reports are often important sources of information about a residency program, they do not in themselves necessarily meet the requirement for a periodic review.

d. Assurance that each residency program establishes and implements formal written criteria and processes for the selection, evaluation, promotion, and dismissal of residents in compliance with both the Institutional and relevant Program Requirements.

e. Assurance of an educational environment in which residents may raise and resolve issues without fear of intimidation or retaliation. This includes:

i. Provision of an organizational system for residents to communicate and exchange information on their working environment and their educational programs. This may be accomplished through a resident organization or other forums in which to address resident issues.

ii. A process by which individual residents can address concerns in a confidential and protected manner.

iii. Establishment and implementation of fair institutional policies and procedures for academic or other disciplinary actions taken against residents.

iv. Establishment and implementation of fair institutional policies and procedures for adjudication of resident complaints and grievances related to actions which could result in dismissal or could significantly threaten a resident's intended career development.

f. Collection of intrainstitutional information and making recommendations on the appropriate funding for resident positions, including benefits and support services.

g. Monitoring of the programs that establish an appropriate work environment and the duty hours of residents.

h. Assurance that the residents' curriculum provides a regular review of ethical, socioeconomic, medical/legal, and cost-containment issues that affect GME and medical practice. The curriculum must also provide an appropriate introduction to communication skills and to research design, statistics, and critical review of the literature necessary for acquiring skills for lifelong learning. There must be appropriate resident participation in departmental scholarly activity, as set forth in the applicable Program Requirements.

INSTITUTIONAL AGREEMENTS

When resident education occurs in a participating institution, the sponsoring institution continues to have responsibility for the quality of that educational experience and must retain authority over the residents' activities. Therefore, current interinstitutional agreements must exist with all of its major participating institutions. The sponsoring institution must ensure that for each accredited program appropriate letters of agreement exist between the sponsoring institution and the participating institution. These agreements should:

1. Identify the officials at the participating institution or facility who will assume administrative, educational, and supervisory responsibility for the resident(s)

2. Outline the educational goals and objectives to be attained within the participating institutions

3. Specify the period of assignment of the residents to the participating institution, the financial arrangements, and the details for insurance and benefits

4. Determine the participating institution's responsibilities for teaching, supervision, and formal evaluation of the residents' performances

5. Establish with the participating institution the policies and procedures that govern the residents' education while rotating to the participating institution.

ACCREDITATION FOR PATIENT CARE

Institutions sponsoring or participating in GME programs should be accredited by the Joint Commission on the Accreditation of Healthcare Organizations (JCAHO), if such institutions are eligible. If an institution is eligible for JCAHO accreditation and chooses not to undergo such accreditation, then the institution should be reviewed by and meet the standards of another recognized body with reasonably equivalent standards. If the institution is not accredited, it must provide a satisfactory explanation of why accreditation has not been either granted or sought.

QUALITY ASSURANCE

Institutions participating in GME must conduct formal quality assurance programs and review complications and deaths.

1. All residents should receive instruction in quality assurance/performance improvement. To the degree possible and in conformance with state law, residents should participate in appropriate components of the institution's performance improvement program.
2. As part of the educational program, it is important that autopsies be performed whenever possible and appropriate. A sufficient number of autopsies representing an adequately diverse spectrum of diseases should be performed to provide an adequate educational experience and to enhance the quality of patient care.
3. Institutions participating in GME must have a medical records system that is available at all times and documents the course of each patient's illness and his or her care.
   The medical records system must be adequate to support the education of residents and quality assurance activities and provide a resource for scholarly activity.

COMPLIANCE WITH ACGME POLICIES AND PROCEDURES

Sponsoring institutions must ensure that their ACGME-accredited programs are in substantial compliance with ACGME policies and procedures as defined in the ACGME Manual of Policies and Procedures for Graduate Medical Education Review Committees. Of particular note are those policies and procedures that govern "Administrative Withdrawal of Accreditation," an action that is not subject to the appeals process:

1. A program may be deemed to have voluntarily withdrawn from the ACGME accreditation process, and an RRC may withdraw accreditation, if the program is not in substantial compliance with:
   a. Site visit and program review policies and procedures;
   b. Directives associated with an accreditation action; or
   c. Requests by the RRC for information.
2. A program that is judged to be delinquent in payment of fees is not eligible for review and will be notified by certified mail, return receipt requested, of the effective date of the withdrawal of accreditation. On that date, the program will be removed from the list of ACGME-accredited programs.

Residents

The sponsoring institution must have written policies and procedures for the recruitment and appointment of residents that comply with the requirements listed below, and it must monitor the compliance of each program with these procedures.

RESIDENT ELIGIBILITY

Applicants with one of the following qualifications are eligible for appointment to accredited residency programs:

1. Graduates of medical schools in the United States and Canada accredited by the Liaison Committee on Medical Education (LCME)
2. Graduates of colleges of osteopathic medicine in the United States accredited by the American Osteopathic Association (AOA)
3. Graduates of medical schools outside the United States and Canada who meet one of the following qualifications:
   a. Have received a currently valid certificate from the Educational Commission for Foreign Medical Graduates, or
   b. Have a full and unrestricted license to practice medicine in a U.S. licensing jurisdiction.
4. Graduates of medical schools outside the United States who have completed a Fifth Pathway program provided by an LCME-accredited medical school. [Note: A Fifth Pathway program is an academic year of supervised clinical education provided by an LCME-accredited medical school to students who meet the following conditions: (1) have completed, in an accredited college or university in the United States, undergraduate premedical education of the quality acceptable for matriculation in an accredited United States Medical school; (2) have studied at a medical school outside the United States and Canada but listed in the World Health Organization Directory of Medical Schools; (3) have completed all of the formal requirements of the foreign medical school except internship and/or social service; (4) have attained a score satisfactory to the sponsoring medical school on a screening examination; and (5) have passed either the Foreign Medical Graduate Examination in the Medical Sciences, Parts I and II of the examination of the National Board of Medical Examiners, or Steps 1 and 2 of the United States Medical Licensing Examination (USMLE).]

Resident Selection

1. The sponsoring institution must ensure that programs select from among eligible applicants on the basis of their preparedness, ability, aptitude, academic credentials, communication skills, and personal qualities such as motivation and integrity. Programs must not discriminate with regard to sex, race, age, religion, color, national origin, disability, or veteran status.
2. In selecting from among qualified applicants, it is strongly suggested that institutions and all of their sponsored programs participate in an organized matching program, where available, such as the National Resident Matching Program (NRMP).

Enrollment of Noneligibles

The enrollment of noneligible residents may be a cause for withdrawal of accreditation of the involved program.

Resident Participation in Educational Activities

Institutions must ensure that residents have the opportunity to:

1. Develop a personal program of learning to foster continued professional growth with guidance from the teaching staff

2. Participate in safe, effective, and compassionate patient care, under supervision, commensurate with their level of advancement and responsibility
3. Participate fully in the educational and scholarly activities of their program and, as required, assume responsibility for teaching and supervising other residents and students
4. Participate as appropriate in institutional programs and medical staff activities and adhere to established practices, procedures, and policies of the institution
5. Participate on appropriate institutional committees and councils whose actions affect their education and /or patient care
6. Submit to the program director or to a designated institutional official at least annually confidential written evaluations of the faculty and of the educational experiences.

Resident Support, Benefits, and Conditions of Employment

Sponsoring and participating institutions should provide all residents with appropriate financial support and benefits. Compensation of residents and distribution of resources for the support of education should be carried out with the advice of the GMEC.

Financial Support

Adequate financial support of residents is necessary to ensure that residents are able to fulfill the responsibilities of their educational programs.

Applicants

Applicants for GME programs must be informed in writing of the terms and conditions of employment and benefits including financial support, vacations, professional leave, parental leave, sick leave, professional liability insurance, hospital and health insurance, disability insurance, and other insurance benefits for the residents and their family, and the conditions under which living quarters, meals, and laundry or their equivalents are to be provided.

Contracts

Sponsoring institutions must provide residents with a written agreement or contract outlining the terms and conditions of their appointment to an educational program, and the institutions must monitor the implementation of these terms and conditions by the program directors. The agreement must contain or reference at least the following:

1. Financial support
2. Vacation policies
3. Professional liability insurance in conformity with the Liability Insurance section just below.
4. Disability insurance and other hospital and health insurance benefits for the residents and their family in conformity with the Disability section just below
5. Professional, parental, and sick-leave benefits in conformity with the Leave of Absence section just below
6. Conditions under which living quarters, meals, and laundry or their equivalents are to be provided

7. Counseling, medical, psychological, and other support services in conformity with the Counseling Services and Physician Impairment sections just below
8. Institutional policies covering sexual and other forms of harassment.

Other Factors

The agreement must also delineate or reference specific policies regarding:
1. Resident's responsibilities
2. Duration of appointment and conditions for reappointment
3. Professional activities outside the educational program
4. Grievance procedures in conformity with the policies described above.

Liability Insurance

Residents in GME must be provided with professional liability coverage for the duration of training. Such coverage must provide legal defense and protection against awards from claims reported or filed after the completion of GME if the alleged acts or omissions of the residents are within the scope of the education program. The coverage to be provided should be consistent with the institution's coverage for other medical/professional practitioners. Each institution must provide current residents and applicants for residency with the details of the institution's professional liability coverage for residents.

Disability Insurance

Institutions sponsoring GME must provide access to insurance, where available, to all residents for disabilities resulting from activities that are part of the educational program.

Leave of Absence

There must be a written institutional policy on leave (with or without pay) for residents that complies with applicable laws. The institution must provide residents with a written policy concerning the effect of leaves of absence, for any reason, on satisfying the criteria for completion of a residency program.

Counseling Services

GME places increasing responsibilities on residents and requires sustained intellectual and physical effort. Therefore, institutions should facilitate resident access to appropriate and confidential counseling, as well as medical and psychological support services.

Physician Impairment

Institutions must have written policies that describe how physician impairment, including that due to substance abuse, will be handled. In addition, institutions should provide an educational program for residents regarding physician impairment, including substance abuse.

Residency Closure/Reduction

If an institution intends to reduce the size of a residency program or to close a residency program, the institution must inform the residents as soon as possible. In the event of such a reduction or closure, institutions must allow residents already in the program to complete their education or assist the residents in enrolling in an ACGME-accredited program in which they can continue their education.

Restrictive Covenants

ACGME-accredited residencies must not require residents to sign a non-competition guarantee.

Resident Supervision, Duty Hours, and Work Environment

Institutions must ensure that their GME programs provide appropriate supervision for all residents, as well as a duty hour schedule and a work environment consistent with proper patient care, the educational needs of residents, and the applicable Program Requirements.

Supervision

There must be sufficient institutional oversight to ensure that residents are appropriately supervised. Residents must be supervised by teaching staff in such a way that the residents assume progressively increasing responsibility according to their level of education, ability, and experience. On-call schedules for teaching staff must be structured to ensure that supervision is readily available to residents on duty. The level of responsibility accorded to each resident must be determined by the teaching staff.

Duty Hours

The sponsoring institution must ensure that each residency program establishes formal policies governing resident duty hours that foster resident education and facilitate the care of patients.

1. The educational goals of the program and learning objectives of residents must not be compromised by excessive reliance on residents to fulfill institutional service obligations. Duty hours, however, must reflect the fact that responsibilities for continuing patient care are not automatically discharged at specific times. Programs must ensure that residents are provided appropriate backup support when patient care responsibilities are especially difficult or prolonged.

2. Resident duty hours and on-call time periods must not be excessive. The structuring of duty hours and on-call schedules must focus on the needs of the patient, continuity of care, and the educational needs of the resident. Duty hours must be consistent with the Institutional and Program Requirements that apply to each program.

3. Work Environment

Sponsoring institutions must provide services and develop systems to minimize the work of residents that is extraneous to their educational programs, ensuring that the following conditions are met:

1. Residents on duty in the hospital must be provided adequate and appropriate food services and sleeping quarters.
2. Patient support services, such as intravenous services, phlebotomy services, and laboratory services, as well as messenger and transporter services, must be provided in a manner appropriate to and consistent with educational objectives and patient care.
3. An effective laboratory, medical records, and radiologic information retrieval system must be in place to provide for appropriate conduct of the educational programs and quality and timely patient care.
4. Appropriate security and personal safety measures must be provided to residents in all locations including but not limited to parking facilities, on-call quarters, hospital and institutional grounds, and related clinical facilities (e.g., medical office building).

2 PROGRAM REQUIREMENTS FOR RESIDENCY EDUCATION IN DIAGNOSTIC RADIOLOGY

Definition and Scope

Diagnostic radiology encompasses a variety of diagnostic and image-guided therapeutic techniques, including all aspects of radiologic diagnosis, nuclear radiology, diagnostic ultrasound, magnetic resonance, computed tomography, interventional procedures, and the use of other forms of radiant energy. The residency program in diagnostic radiology shall offer a quality graduate medical educational experience of adequate scope and depth in all these associated diagnostic disciplines.

Duration and Scope of Education

Resident education in diagnostic radiology must include 5 years of clinically oriented graduate medical education, of which 4 years must be in diagnostic radiology. The clinical year must consist of ACGME or equivalent accredited training in internal medicine, pediatrics, surgery or surgical specialties, obstetrics and gynecology, neurology, family practice, emergency medicine, or any combination of these, or an ACGME or equivalent accredited transitional year.

Source: ACGME, June 22, 1998; effective, July 1, 1999. *Graduate Medical Education Directory, 2001–2002*, American Medical Association.

If the clinical year is offered by the institution of the core residency, and it is not itself an ACGME accredited year, the program director will be responsible for assuring the quality of the year. The clinical year should be completed within the first 24 months of training.

The diagnostic radiology program shall offer a minimum of 4 years of graduate medical education (including vacation and meeting time) in diagnostic radiology, of which at least 42 months of training must be in the parent or integrated institution(s). [Note: Time spent attending the Armed Forces Institute of Pathology (AFIP) course is excluded.] The minimum period of training in nuclear radiology shall be 6 months. The maximum period of training in any subspecialty area shall be 12 months.

Institutional Organization

All educational components of a residency program should be related to program goals. The program design and structure must be approved by the RRC as part of the regular review process.

SPONSORING INSTITUTION

The residency program in diagnostic radiology must have one parent institution with primary responsibility for the entire program. When any institution(s) other than the parent is utilized for the clinical or basic science education of a resident in diagnostic radiology, letters of agreement must be provided by the appropriate institutional authority.

The institution must demonstrate commitment to the program in terms of financial and academic support, including the timely appointment of a permanent department chair.

PARTICIPATING INSTITUTIONS

Institutions may participate on an affiliated or an integrated basis. An accredited program may be independent or may occur in two or more institutions that develop formal agreements and conjoint responsibilities to provide complementary facilities, teaching staff, and teaching sessions. When another institution is utilized and a single program director assumes responsibility for the entire residency, including the appointment of all residents and teaching staff, that institution is designated as integrated. Within a single program some participating hospitals may qualify as integrated, whereas others are merely affiliated. Rotations to affiliated institutions may not exceed 6 months during the 4 years of training. [Note: Time spent attending the AFIP course is excluded] Rotations to integrated institutions are not limited in duration. Participation by any affiliated institution providing more than 3 months of training must be approved by the RRC. Prior approval of the RRC must be obtained for participation of an institution on an integrated basis, regardless of the duration of the rotations.

The purpose of another institution's participation and the educational contribution to the total training program shall be defined. Service responsibility alone at a participating institution does not constitute a suitable educational experience. Affiliation shall be avoided with institutions that are at such a distance from the parent institution as to make resident attendance at rounds and conferences impractical, unless there is a comparable educational experience at the affiliated institution.

APPOINTMENT OF RESIDENTS

Peer contact and discussion are as important to the learning process as contact with teaching faculty. The number of diagnostic radiology residents in the program must be sufficient to provide for frequent and meaningful discussion with peers as well as to provide appropriate coverage for adequate patient care. Appointment of a minimum of eight residents with, on average, two appointed each year, is required for an efficient learning environment. Prior approval by the RRC is required for an increase in the number of residents.

The complement of residents must be commensurate with the total capacity of the program to offer an adequate educational experience in diagnostic radiology. A reasonable volume is no less than 7000 radiologic examinations per year per resident. The number of examinations in each of the subspecialty areas must be of sufficient volume to ensure adequate training experience.

Faculty Qualifications and Responsibilities

The program director and teaching faculty are responsible for the general administration of a program, including those activities related to the recruitment, selection, instruction, supervision, counseling, evaluation, and advancement of residents and the maintenance of records related to program accreditation.

PROGRAM DIRECTOR
Qualifications

1. There must be a single program director responsible for the program. The program director must be a faculty member who is a diagnostic radiologist and must contribute sufficient time to the program to fulfill all the responsibilities inherent in meeting the educational goals of the program. The program director must have appropriate authority to organize and fulfill administrative and teaching responsibilities to achieve the educational goals.

2. The program director must be licensed to practice medicine in the state where the institution that sponsors the program is located. (Certain federal programs are exempted.)

3. The program director shall be certified by the American Board of Radiology or possess suitable equivalent qualifications, as determined by the RRC.

4. The program director also must hold an appointment in good standing to the medical staff of an institution participating in the program. A complete curriculum vitae of the program director shall be filed with the Executive Director of the RRC at the time of appointment and updated with each review of the program by the RRC.

5. The program director should have sufficient academic and administrative experience to ensure effective implementation of these Program Requirements and should have at least 3 years of participation as an active faculty member in an accredited residency program.

Responsibilities

The program director shall be responsible for the total training in diagnostic radiology, which includes the instruction and supervision of residents. The program director shall be responsible for evaluation of the teaching faculty in concert with the department chair. The program director is responsible for promptly notifying the Executive Director of the RRC in writing of any major changes in the program, including changes in leadership. Prior approval of the RRC is required for the addition or deletion of a major participating hospital, for an increase in the number of residents in the program, and for a major change in the format of the program. On review of a proposal for major change in a program, the RRC may determine that a site visit is necessary.

The program director is also responsible for the following:

1. Preparation of a written statement outlining the curriculum and educational goals and objectives of the program with respect to knowledge, skills, and other attributes of residents at each level of training and for each major rotation or other program assignment. This statement must be distributed to residents and members of the teaching faculty. It should be readily available for review.
2. Selection of residents for appointment to the program in accordance with institutional and departmental policies and procedures.
3. Selection and supervision of resident rotations, teaching faculty from the department professional staff, and other program personnel at each institution participating in the program.
4. Supervision of residents through explicit written descriptions of supervisory lines of responsibility for the care of patients. Such guidelines must be communicated to all members of the program faculty. Residents must be provided with prompt, reliable systems for communication and interaction with supervisory physicians.
5. Implementation of fair procedures, as established by the sponsoring institution, regarding academic discipline and resident complaints or grievances.
6. Preparation of an accurate statistical and narrative description of the program as requested by the RRC.
7. Monitoring of resident stress, including mental or emotional conditions and drug-or alcohol-related dysfunction, inhibiting performance or learning. The program director and teaching faculty should be sensitive to the need for timely provision of confidential counseling and psychological support services to residents. Training situations that consistently produce undesirable stress on residents must be evaluated and modified.

Faculty

1. All members of the teaching faculty must demonstrate a strong interest in the education of residents, sound clinical and teaching abilities, support of the goals and objectives of the program, a commitment to their own continuing medical education, and participation in scholarly activities. There must be a sufficient number of teaching faculty. At a minimum, there must be one full-time equivalent physician faculty member at the parent and integrated institutions for every resident in training, in the program. The teaching faculty must be qualified in those areas in which they are assigned to instruct and supervise residents, and they must contribute sufficient time to the program to provide adequate instruction and supervision.
2. Didactic and clinical teaching must be provided by faculty with documented interests and expertise in the subspecialty involved. The teaching faculty responsible for the training in each designated subspecialty area must demonstrate a commitment to the subspecialty. Such commitment may be demonstrated by any of the following: (1) fellowship training or 3 years of subspecialty practice, (2) membership in a subspecialty society, (3) publications and presentations in the subspecialty, and (4) annual continuing medical education (CME) credits in the subspecialty.
3. At least one faculty member must be designated to have primary responsibility for the educational content of each of the nine subspecialty areas. This individual must practice at least 50% of his or her time in the department. The nine subspecialty areas are neuroradiology, musculoskeletal radiology, vascular and interventional radiology, chest radiology, breast imaging, abdominal radiology, pediatric radiology, ultrasonography (including obstetrical and vascular ultrasound), and nuclear radiology. No faculty member can have primary responsibility for the educational content of more than one subspecialty area, although faculty can have clinical responsibility and/or teaching responsibilities in several subspecialty areas. A pediatric radiologist may have a primary appointment at another institution and still be the designated faculty member supervising pediatric radiologic education.
4. A member of the teaching faculty of each participating institution must be designated to assume responsibility for the day-to-day activities of the program at that institution, with overall coordination by the program director.
5. The teaching faculty must be organized and have regular documented meetings to review program goals and objectives as well as program effectiveness in achieving them. At least one resident representative should participate in these reviews. The faculty should evaluate the utilization of the resources available to the program, the contribution of each institution participating in the program, the financial and administrative support of the program, the volume and variety of patients available to the program for educational purposes, the performance of members of the teaching faculty, and the quality of supervision of residents.

Other Program Personnel

Programs must be provided with the additional professional, technical, and clerical personnel needed to support the administration and educational conduct of the program.

Facilities and Resources

1. The program must provide not only adequate space, equipment, and other pertinent facilities to ensure an effective educational experience for residents in diagnostic radiology but also the modern facilities and equipment required in all of the subspecialty rotations.
2. There must be 24-hour access to an on-site departmental library or to a collection of journals, references, and resource

materials pertinent to progressive levels of education in diagnostic radiology and associated fields in each institution participating in a residency program. On-site libraries and/or collections of texts and journals must include standard diagnostic radiology and radiologic subspecialty textbooks and major radiology journals.

3. Residents must have ready access to a major medical library, either at the institution where the residents are located or through arrangement with convenient nearby institutions. The institutional library must have facilities for electronic retrieval of information from medical databases and on-line literature searches.

4. Service commitments must not compromise the achievement of the program's educational goals and objectives.

The Educational Program

CLINICAL COMPONENTS

The program in diagnostic radiology must provide a sufficient volume and variety of patients to ensure that residents gain experience in the full range of radiologic examinations, procedures, and interpretations. A reasonable volume is no less than 75,000 total radiologic examinations at the parent or integrated program and no less than 7000 radiologic examinations per year per resident. The number of examinations in each of the subspecialty areas must be of sufficient volume to ensure adequate training experience. If volume in any subspecialty area is less than acceptable, a plan must be developed to increase trainee exposure. The presence of residents and subspecialty residents from outside institutions for limited rotations should not dilute the educational experience of the core program residents.

The clinical training must provide for progressive, supervised responsibility for patient care and must ensure that the supervised resident performs those procedures commonly accepted in all aspects of diagnostic radiology. The training must include progressive study and experience in all of the diagnostic radiologic subspecialties. The training program should ensure sufficient time to gain experience in neuroradiology, musculoskeletal radiology, vascular and interventional radiology, chest radiology, breast imaging, abdominal radiology, pediatric radiology, ultrasonography (including obstetrical and vascular ultrasound), and nuclear radiology. Additionally, each resident must have documented supervised experience in interventional procedures, for example, image-guided biopsies, drainage procedures, noncoronary angioplasty, embolization and infusion procedures, and percutaneous introduction techniques.

The program director must require that residents maintain a record (electronic or written) in which they document the performance, interpretation, and complications of vascular, interventional, and invasive procedures. The record must be reviewed by the program director or faculty designee on a yearly basis.

Training and experience are required in plain film interpretation, computed tomography, magnetic resonance imaging, ultrasonography, angiography, and nuclear radiology examinations related to cardiovascular disease. The program must also provide instruction in cardiac anatomy, physiology, and pathology, including the coronary arteries, as essential to the interpretation of cardiac imaging studies. This training must include both the adult and the pediatric age group. Radiologic education in different organ systems must provide the opportunity for residents to develop adequate knowledge regarding normal and pathologic physiology, including the biologic and pharmacologic actions of materials administered to patients in diagnostic studies.

Each resident must have basic life-support training, and advanced cardiac life-support training is recommended.

DIDACTIC COMPONENTS

The education in diagnostic radiology must occur in an environment that encourages the interchange of knowledge and experience among residents in the program and with residents in other major clinical specialties located in those institutions participating in the program.

Diagnostic radiologic physics, radiation biology, radiation protection, and pathology are required elements of the curriculum. In view of the importance of understanding pathology as a basis for radiologic diagnosis, emphasis should be placed on its study. Radiologic/pathologic conferences are required for those residents who do not participate in formalized extramural pathology teaching programs.

Computer applications in radiology, practice management, and health systems and quality improvement are also required curriculum components.

Teaching files (electronic or film) of cases related to all aspects of diagnostic radiology must be available for use by residents. Aggregates of these files should contain a minimum of 1000 cases that are actively maintained and continually enhanced with new cases. The American College of Radiology learning file or its equivalent should be available to residents; this only partially meets the teaching file requirements.

Conferences and teaching rounds must be correlated and provide for progressive resident participation. There should be intradepartmental conferences as well as interdepartmental conferences of appropriate frequency with each major clinical department in which both residents and faculty participate on a regular basis.

RESIDENT POLICIES

Supervision

The responsibility or independence given to residents should depend on their knowledge, manual skill, and experience. Faculty supervision must be available at all sites of training. The resident in the first year of training in the diagnostic radiology program must have a minimum of 6 months of training in diagnostic radiology prior to independent in-house on-call responsibilities. Residents must always have faculty backup when taking night or weekend call. All radiologic images must be reviewed, and all reports must be signed by faculty.

Duty Hours and Conditions of Work

Duty hours and night and weekend call for residents must reflect the concept of responsibility for adequate patient care.

However, residents must not be required regularly to perform excessively difficult or prolonged duties. It is recommended that residents should be allowed to spend at least 1 full day out of 7 away from the hospital and should be assigned on-call duty in the hospital no more than, on average, every third night. It is the responsibility of the program director to monitor resident assignments to ensure adherence to this recommendation.

OTHER REQUIRED COMPONENTS

Scholarly Activity

Graduate medical education must take place in an environment of inquiry and scholarship in which residents participate in the development of new knowledge, learn to evaluate research findings, and develop habits of inquiry as a continuing professional responsibility. The responsibility for establishing and maintaining an environment of inquiry and scholarship rests with the teaching faculty. Although not all members of a teaching faculty must be investigators, the faculty as a whole must demonstrate broad involvement in scholarly activity. This activity should include:

1. Active participation of the teaching faculty in clinical discussions, rounds, and conferences in a manner that promotes a spirit of inquiry and scholarship. Scholarship implies an in-depth understanding of basic mechanisms of normal and abnormal states and the application of current knowledge to practice.
2. Participation in journal clubs and research conferences.
3. Active participation in regional or national professional and scientific societies, particularly through presentations at the organizations' meetings and publication in their journals.
4. Participation in CME programs.
5. Participation in research, particularly in projects that are funded following peer review and/or result in publication or presentations at regional and national scientific meetings.
6. Offering of guidance and technical support (e.g., research design, statistical analysis) for residents involved in scholarly activities.

Resident Research

During their training, all residents should be encouraged to engage in an investigative project under faculty supervision. This may take the form of laboratory research, clinical research, or the retrospective analysis of data from patients; results of such projects shall be suitable for publication or presentation at local, regional, or national scientific meetings.

Evaluation

RESIDENT EVALUATION

The program director is responsible for regular evaluation of residents' knowledge, skills, and overall performance, includ-

ing the development of professional attitudes consistent with being a physician. Evaluations of each resident's progress and competence should be conducted preferably at the end of each rotation, but not less than four times yearly. The evaluation must concern itself with intellectual abilities, attitudes, character skills, and clinical and technical competence. The program director or the program director's designee must meet with all the residents at least semiannually to discuss these evaluations and provide feedback on performance. More frequent reviews of performance for residents experiencing difficulties or receiving unfavorable evaluations are required. There must be provision for appropriate and timely feedback of the content of all evaluations to the resident. Residents should be advanced to positions of higher responsibility only on the basis of their satisfactory progressive scholarship and professional growth. The program must maintain a permanent record of the evaluation and counseling process for each resident. Such records must be accessible to the resident and other authorized personnel.

There must be a written final evaluation for each resident who completes the program. The evaluation must include a review of the resident's performance during the final period of training and should verify that the resident has demonstrated sufficient professional ability to practice competently and independently. The final evaluation should be part of the resident's permanent record maintained by the institution.

FACULTY AND PROGRAM EVALUATION

The program must provide the opportunity for residents to provide written confidential evaluation of the faculty and the program at least annually. Each faculty member must review his or her evaluations.

The educational effectiveness of a program must be evaluated in a systematic manner. In particular, the quality of the curriculum and the extent to which the educational goals have been met by residents must be assessed. Anonymous written evaluations by residents should be utilized in this process.

Board Certification

The RRC will consider the performance of a program's graduates on the examinations of the American Board of Radiology as one measure of the quality of the training program. During the most recent 5-year period, at least 50% of its graduates should pass without condition the written and oral examinations on the first attempt.

Residents who plan to seek certification by the American Board of Radiology should communicate with the Executive Director of the Board to be certain of all requirements, including duration of training, for admission to the examination process.

3 POLICIES AND PROCEDURES FOR RESIDENCY EDUCATION IN THE SUBSPECIALTIES OF DIAGNOSTIC RADIOLOGY

Subspecialty programs must be administratively linked to an accredited core residency program in diagnostic radiology. (The only exception is pediatric radiology, as discussed below.) An application for accreditation of a new subspecialty program will be considered only if the core program has full accreditation. An application will not be accepted for review if the core program in diagnostic radiology is accredited on a provisional or a probationary basis, or if it has been accredited with a warning that adverse action will be taken if it is not in substantial compliance with the Essentials of Accredited Residencies in Graduate Medical Education at the time of the next review.

A subspecialty program in pediatric radiology may not necessarily be administratively linked to an accredited core residency program in diagnostic radiology if the pediatric radiology program is conducted in a children's hospital. In such a case, the subspecialty program may be considered free standing and therefore not required to be under the sponsorship of a diagnostic radiology residency program.

An on-site survey of the proposed program is required for the initial review by the Residency Review Committee. Accreditation will be granted on the basis of the application and the written report from the on-site survey of the proposed program. Following the initial approval, the subspecialty program will be surveyed and reviewed in conjunction with the core diagnostic radiology program.

Subspecialty programs will be designated as "accredited" or "non-accredited." No other delineation of accreditation categories will be used. The accreditation status of the subspecialty program will be directly related to that of the core diagnostic radiology program, as follows:

1. Subspecialty programs may be cited for deficiencies and advised that either the deficiencies must be corrected by the specified time or accreditation will be withdrawn regardless of the accreditation status of the associated diagnostic radiology program.
2. If the associated diagnostic radiology program is accredited on a probationary basis, or accredited with a warning that adverse action will be taken, the subspecialty program will be informed that its accreditation status is also in jeopardy. Thereafter, accreditation of the subspecialty programs will be withdrawn if the RRC finds that the sponsoring institution(s) is (are) not making satisfactory progress in addressing the adverse accreditation status of the core diagnostic radiology program.
3. Withdrawal of accreditation of the core diagnostic radiology residency program will result in simultaneous withdrawal of accreditation of the subspecialty program.
4. In the case of withholding of accreditation or withdrawing accreditation of subspecialty programs, the Procedures for Proposed Adverse Actions and the Procedures for Appeal of Adverse Actions apply.

Source: ACGME, June 22, 1998; effective, July 1, 1999. *Graduate Medical Education Directory, 2001–2002*, American Medical Association.

4 PROGRAM REQUIREMENTS FOR RESIDENCY EDUCATION IN THE SUBSPECIALTIES OF DIAGNOSTIC RADIOLOGY

These requirements apply to all the accredited subspecialty areas and should be consulted with the individual subspecialty Program Requirements.

General Information

1. A residency education program in a subspecialty of diagnostic radiology is an educational experience of at least 1 year designed to develop advanced knowledge and skills in a specific clinical area. All educational components of the program should be related to program goals. The program design and/or structure must be approved by the RRC as part of the regular review process.

Completion of an ACGME-accredited diagnostic radiology residency or its equivalent is a prerequisite for entry into a subspecialty program of diagnostic radiology.
2. Residency education programs in the subspecialties of diagnostic radiology may be accredited only in institutions that either sponsor a residency education program in diagnostic radiology accredited by the ACGME or are integrated by formal agreement into such programs (*see* Program Requirements for Pediatric Radiology section, below, for exceptions to this requirement.) Close cooperation between the subspecialty and residency program directors is required.
3. Rotations to affiliated institutions can be approved for a period not exceeding 25% of the total program; adequate educational

Source: ACGME, February, 1994; effective, January, 1995. *Graduate Medical Education Directory 2001–2002*, American Medical Association.

justification for such rotations must be provided to the RRC prior to implementation. The definitions governing affiliated and integrated institutions in the Program Requirements for Residency Education in Diagnostic Radiology also apply to the subspecialty programs of diagnostic radiology.

4. Subspecialty programs will not be approved if they have substantial negative impact on the education of the diagnostic radiology residents in the core program.

Faculty Qualifications and Responsibilities

The program director and faculty are responsible for the general administration of a program, including activities related to the recruitment, selection, supervision, counseling, evaluation, and advancement of residents and the maintenance of records related to program accreditation. Subspecialty education programs must provide a scholarly environment for acquiring the necessary cognitive and procedural clinical skills essential to the practice of the specific subspecialty. This objective can be achieved only when the program director, the supporting faculty and staff, and the administration are fully committed to the educational program. It is also imperative that appropriate resources and facilities be present. Service obligations must not compromise educational goals and objectives.

QUALIFICATIONS OF THE PROGRAM DIRECTOR

There must be a single program director responsible for the subspecialty program. The director must be an experienced educator and supervisor of residents in the subspecialty. He or she must be certified by the American Board of Radiology in diagnostic radiology or radiology or possess equivalent qualifications and shall have had postresidency experience in the subspecialty, preferably fellowship training (see Program Requirements for Residency Education in the individual subspecialties for subspecialty certification requirements.) The program director must be licensed to practice medicine in the state where the institution that sponsors the program is located. (Certain federal programs are exempted.) The program director must be a member of the radiology faculty, spend essentially all professional time in the subspecialty, and devote sufficient time to fulfill all responsibilities inherent in meeting the educational goals of the program.

RESPONSIBILITIES OF THE PROGRAM DIRECTOR

It is the responsibility of the subspecialty program director to support the residency education program by devoting his or her principal effort to its management and administration, as well as to teaching, research, and clinical care limited to the integrated institutions. This general responsibility includes the following specifics:

1. Preparation of a written statement outlining the educational goals of the program with respect to knowledge, skills, and other attributes of residents and for each major rotation or other program assignment. This statement must be distributed to residents and members of the teaching staff and should be readily available for review.

2. Selection of residents for appointment to the program in accordance with institutional and departmental policies and procedures.

3. Selection and supervision of the teaching staff and other program personnel at each institution participating in the program.

4. Supervision of residents through explicit written descriptions of supervisory lines of responsibility for the care of patients. Such guidelines must be communicated to all members of the program staff. Residents must be provided with prompt, reliable systems for communication and interaction with supervisory physicians.

5. Regular evaluation of residents' knowledge, skills, and overall performance, including the development of professional attitudes consistent with being a physician.

6. Implementation of fair procedures, as established by the sponsoring institution, regarding academic discipline and resident complaints or grievances.

7. Monitoring of resident stress, including mental or emotional conditions inhibiting performance or learning and drug- or alcohol-related dysfunction. Program directors and teaching staff should be sensitive to the need for timely provision of confidential counseling and psychological support services to residents. Training situations that consistently produce undesirable stress on residents must be evaluated and modified.

8. Preparation of an accurate statistical and narrative description of the program.

9. Notification of the RRC regarding major programmatic changes. Prior approval of the RRC is required for the addition or deletion of a major participating hospital, for an increase in the number of residents in the program, and for a major change in the program's organization.

FACULTY

There must be a sufficient number of teaching staff with documented qualifications to instruct and supervise adequately all the residents in the program. Members of the teaching staff must be able to devote sufficient time to meet their supervisory and teaching responsibilities.

All members of the teaching staff must demonstrate a strong interest in the education of residents, have sound clinical and teaching abilities, support the goals and objectives of the program, have a commitment to their own continuing medical education, and participate in scholarly activities.

A member of the teaching staff of each participating institution must be designated to assume responsibility for the day-to-day activities of the program at that institution, with overall coordination by the program director. The teaching staff must be organized and have regular documented meetings to review program goals and objectives as well as program effectiveness in achieving them. At least one resident representative should participate in these reviews.

The teaching staff should periodically evaluate the utilization of the resources available to the program, the contribution of each institution participating in the program, the financial and administrative support of the program, the volume and variety of patients available to the program for educational purposes, the performance of members of the teaching staff, and the quality of supervision of residents.

OTHER PROGRAM PERSONNEL

Programs must be provided with the additional professional, technical, and clerical personnel needed to support the administration and educational conduct of the program.

Facilities and Resources

SPACE AND EQUIPMENT

See Program Requirements for Residency Education in the individual subspecialties for space and equipment requirements.

LIBRARY

Residents must have ready access to a major medical library, either at the institution where the residents are located or through arrangement with convenient nearby institutions. There must be access to an on-site library or to a collection of appropriate texts and journals in each institution participating in a residency program. Access to computerized literature search facilities is necessary. On-site libraries and/or collections of texts and journals must be readily available during nights and weekends.

Educational Program

The director and teaching staff must prepare and comply with written goals for the program. All educational components of the program should be related to the program goals. The program design must be approved by the RRC as part of the regular review process. A written statement of the educational objectives must be given to each resident.

A postgraduate residency must provide advanced education so that the residents can acquire special skill and knowledge in a specific subspecialty. This education should consist of a cognitive and a technical component. The cognitive component should emphasize the scholarly attributes of self-instruction, teaching, skilled clinical analysis, sound judgment, and research creativity. The technical component must provide appropriate opportunity for the residents to acquire the operative and other psychomotor skills required for the practice of the subspecialty.

CLINICAL COMPONENTS

A sufficient number of patients must be available to ensure appropriate inpatient and outpatient experience for each subspecialty resident without adversely affecting the experience of residents in the diagnostic radiology core program.

The total number of residents is dependent on the program's resources and its capacity to provide an excellent educational experience.

DIDACTIC COMPONENTS

Subspecialty conferences, including review of all current complications and deaths, seminars, and clinical and basic science instruction, must be regularly scheduled. Active participation of the subspecialty resident in the planning and the production of these meetings is essential.

SUPERVISION

A resident must have the opportunity to provide consultation with faculty supervision. He or she should have clearly defined educational responsibilities for diagnostic radiology residents, medical students, and professional personnel. These teaching experiences should correlate basic biomedical knowledge with the clinical aspects of the subspecialty.

There must be close interaction between the core residency program in diagnostic radiology and the subspecialty program. Lines of responsibility for the diagnostic radiology residents and the subspecialty resident must be clearly defined. It is imperative that the educational program for the subspecialty resident not adversely affect the education of the diagnostic radiology residents, in terms of either experience or patient responsibility.

DUTY HOURS AND CONDITIONS OF WORK

The program director must establish an environment that is optimal both for resident education and for patient care, including the responsibility for continuity of care, while ensuring that undue stress and fatigue among residents are avoided. It is the program director's responsibility to ensure assignment of appropriate in-hospital duty hours so that residents are not subjected to excessively difficult or prolonged working hours. It is desirable that residents' work schedules be designed so that on average, excluding exceptional patient care needs, residents have at least 1 day out of 7 free of routine responsibilities and be on call in the hospital no more often than every third night.

During the on-call hours residents should be provided with adequate sleeping, lounge, and food facilities. There must be adequate backup so that patient care is not jeopardized during or following assigned periods of duty. Support services and systems must be such that the resident does not spend an inordinate amount of time in noneducational activities that can be discharged properly by other personnel.

SCHOLARLY ACTIVITY

Graduate medical education must take place in an environment of inquiry and scholarship in which residents participate in the development of new knowledge, learn to evaluate research findings, and develop habits of inquiry as a continuing professional responsibility. The responsibility for establishing and maintaining an environment of inquiry and scholarship rests with the teaching staff. Although not all members of a teaching staff must be investigators, the staff as a whole must demonstrate broad involvement in scholarly activity. This activity should include

1. Active participation of the teaching staff in clinical discussions, rounds, and conferences in a manner that promotes a spirit of inquiry and scholarship. Scholarship implies an in-depth understanding of basic mechanisms of normal and abnormal states and the application of current knowledge to practice
2. Participation in journal clubs and research conferences
3. Active participation in regional or national professional and scientific societies, particularly through presentations at the organizations' meetings and publications in their journals

4. Participation in research, particularly in projects that are funded following peer review and/or result in publications or presentations at regional and national scientific meetings

5. Offering of guidance and technical support (e.g., research design, statistical analysis) for residents involved in research

6. Provision of support for resident participation in scholarly activities.

RESEARCH

A subspecialty program should have an investigational component such that the residents may become familiar with the design, implementation, and interpretation of clinical research studies. Facilities should be made available for research activity (*see* Program Requirements for the individual subspecialties for further requirements).

Evaluation
RESIDENTS

Subspecialty program directors must establish clearly defined procedures for regular evaluation of residents' knowledge, skills, and overall performance, including the development of professional attitudes consistent with being a physician. The assessment must include cognitive, motor, and interpersonal skills as well as judgment.

The program director, with participation of members of the teaching staff, shall:

1. At least semiannually evaluate the knowledge, skills, and professional growth of the residents, using appropriate criteria and procedures

2. Communicate each evaluation to the resident in a timely manner

3. Advance residents to positions of higher responsibility only on the basis of evidence of their satisfactory progressive scholarship and professional growth

4. Maintain a permanent record of evaluation for each resident and have it accessible to the resident and other authorized personnel

5. Provide a written final evaluation for each resident who completes the program. The evaluation must include a review of the resident's performance during the final period of training and should verify that the resident has demonstrated sufficient professional ability to practice competently and independently. This final evaluation should be part of the resident's permanent record maintained by the institution.

FACULTY

Faculty must be evaluated at least annually to review teaching abilities, commitment to the educational program, clinical knowledge, and scholarly activities. Residents should participate in these evaluations.

PROGRAM

The educational effectiveness of a program must be evaluated in a systematic manner. In particular, the quality of the curriculum and the extent to which the educational goals have been met by residents must be assessed by the subspecialty program director, the core diagnostic radiology program director, and the Institutional Review Committee on a regular basis. Written evaluations by residents should be utilized in this process.

Board Certification

Residents who plan to seek certification by the American Board of Radiology should communicate with the Executive Director of the Board to ascertain the current requirements for acceptance as a candidate for subspecialty certification.

5 PROGRAM REQUIREMENTS FOR RESIDENT EDUCATION IN ABDOMINAL RADIOLOGY

In addition to complying with the Program Requirements for Residency Education in the Subspecialties of Diagnostic Radiology, programs must comply with the following requirements, which in some cases may exceed the common requirements.

Scope and Duration of Training
DEFINITION AND SCOPE OF THE SPECIALTY

Abdominal radiology constitutes the application and interpretation of conventional radiology, computed tomography, ultrasonography, magnetic resonance imaging, nuclear medicine, fluoroscopy, and interventional methods customarily included within the specialty of diagnostic radiology as they apply to dis-

eases involving the gastrointestinal tract, the genitourinary tract, and the intraperitoneal and extraperitoneal abdominal organs.

The program must be organized to substantially enhance the residents' knowledge of the application of all forms of diagnostic imaging and interventional techniques to the unique clinical pathophysiologic problems encountered in diseases affecting the gastrointestinal and genitourinary systems. The program should include education in normal and pathologic anatomy and physiology of gastrointestinal and genitourinary disease and be structured to develop expertise in the appropriate application of all forms of diagnostic imaging and interventions to problems of the abdomen and pelvis.

Source: ACGME, June, 1998; Effective, June, 1998. *Graduate Medical Education Directory, 2001–2002*. American Medical Association.

DURATION OF TRAINING

The program shall offer 1 year of graduate medical education in abdominal radiology. This year of training must follow successful completion of an ACGME-accredited program in diagnostic radiology or its equivalent.

Faculty Qualifications and Responsibilities

The director of the program in abdominal radiology must be an experienced educator and supervisor of residents in abdominal radiology. The program director must be certified by the American Board of Radiology in radiology or diagnostic radiology, or possess equivalent qualifications, and shall have had postresidency experience in abdominal radiology, preferably fellowship training.

The faculty should include, in addition to the program director, at least one other full-time radiologist specializing in abdominal radiology. At a minimum, the program faculty must have two full-time equivalent faculty members dedicated to the program. Although it is desirable that abdominal radiologists supervise special imaging such as computed tomography, ultrasonography, and magnetic resonance imaging, when they are not expert in a special imaging technique, other radiologists who are specialists in those areas must be part-time members of the abdominal radiology faculty. The faculty must provide didactic teaching and supervision of the residents' performance and interpretation of all abdominal imaging procedures (*see* Program Requirements for the Subspecialties of Diagnostic Radiology for additional program director and faculty requirements).

The total number of residents in the program must be commensurate with the capacity of the program to offer an adequate educational experience in abdominal radiology. The minimum number of residents need not be greater than one, but at least two residents is desirable. To ensure adequate supervision and evaluation of the residents' academic progress, the faculty/resident ratio should not be less than one faculty member to each resident.

Facilities and Resources

SPACE AND EQUIPMENT

Modern imaging equipment and adequate space must be available to accomplish the overall educational program in abdominal radiology. There must be state-of-the-art equipment for conventional radiography, digital fluoroscopy, computed tomography, ultrasonography, nuclear medicine, and magnetic resonance imaging. Laboratory and pathology services must be adequate to support the educational experience in abdominal radiology. Adequate areas for display of images, interpretation of images, and consultation with clinicians must be available.

LIBRARY

Ancillary teaching resources must include access to a medical library. A variety of textbooks, journals, and other teaching materials in abdominal radiology and related medical and surgical fields must be available. A subspecialty teaching file and in-house file must be actively developed and available for use by residents. The American College of Radiology teaching files in gastrointestinal and genitourinary radiology only partially meet this requirement.

Educational Program

CLINICAL COMPONENTS

The program must provide both clinical and didactic experiences that encompass the full breadth of diseases and their pathophysiology, with coverage of uncommon problems involving the gastrointestinal tract, genitourinary tract, and abdomen, including but not limited to the liver and biliary system, pancreas, stomach, esophagus, small bowel, colon, spleen, kidneys, adrenal glands, bladder, male and female reproductive systems, and lymphatic system.

The program must provide an adequate volume and variety of imaging studies and interventional procedures and must provide instruction in their indications, appropriate utilization, risks, and alternatives. The resident must have the opportunity to perform the abdominal imaging studies, including urethrography, urography, cystography, hysterosalpingography, computed tomography, ultrasonography, magnetic resonance imaging, and plain radiographic and fluoroscopic studies of the hollow gastrointestinal tract.

The resident also must gain experience in performing guided biopsies of intraperitoneal and retroperitoneal structures as well as aspiration and drainage of abscesses. The resident must be familiar with the indications and complications of percutaneous nephrostomy and transhepatic cholangiography and must obtain experience in providing fluoroscopic guidance for the dilation of gastrointestinal, biliary, pancreatic, and ureteric duct strictures. Interpretation of endoscopic retrograde cholangiopancreatography (ERCP) and operative cholangiography must be taught. The program also should provide opportunity, through conferences and individual consultation, for the residents to integrate invasive procedures, when indicated, into optimal care plans for patients, even though formal responsibility for performing the procedures may not be part of the program.

The program must provide instruction in the indications for, as well as the complications of, certain procedures, such as visceral angiography, tumor embolization, radionuclide scintigraphy, lithotripsy, gastrostomy, nephrostomy, and cholecystostomy.

Graded responsibility or independence given to residents should depend on their knowledge, technical skill, and experience. Attending faculty must be available to perform and/or supervise procedures as required.

DIDACTIC COMPONENTS

A major goal of the didactic portion of the training program should be to provide the resident with an understanding of the pathophysiology of diseases that affect the gastrointestinal and genitourinary tracts. Diagnostic skill and understanding of uncommon problems in abdominal disease (as well as of the indications, risks, limitations, alternatives, and appropriate utilization of imaging and interventional procedures) should be part of the body of knowledge imparted. Education must be available in the basic radiologic sciences, e.g., diagnostic radiologic physics, radiation biology, and the pharmacology of radiographic contrast materials.

There must be intradepartmental conferences, as well as conferences with related clinical departments, in which residents in abdominal radiology participate on a regular basis. These should include one or more weekly departmental conferences in abdominal radiology and at least one monthly interdepartmental clinical conference.

Residents must be given the opportunity to present the radiologic aspects of cases in combined clinical conferences related to allied disciplines. They also should prepare clinically and/or pathologically proven cases for inclusion in an ongoing teaching file. There must be daily image interpretation sessions requiring that residents reach their own diagnostic conclusions, which are then reviewed and critiqued by faculty. Diagnostic reports generated by residents should be closely reviewed for content, level of confidence, grammar, and style.

Residents should be encouraged to attend and participate in regional conferences. They should attend at least one national meeting or postgraduate course in abdominal radiology during the year of fellowship training.

ADDITIONAL REQUIRED COMPONENTS

There should be an ACGME-accredited residency or subspecialty training program available in general surgery, gas-

troenterology, oncology, urology, gynecology, and pathology; at a minimum, there must be Board-certified (or equivalent) specialists in these areas to provide appropriate patient populations and educational resources in the institution. These specialists may serve as additional faculty.

SCHOLARLY ACTIVITIES

The training program should have a research component that offers an opportunity for residents to learn the fundamentals of design, performance, and interpretation of research studies, as well as how to evaluate investigative methods. Particular attention should be given to developing competence in critical assessment of new imaging modalities and of the radiologic literature, and residents will be expected to participate actively in research projects. The program must provide sufficient office space, supplies, and secretarial support to enable residents to conduct research projects as well as perform literature searches, manuscript preparation, statistical analysis, and photography.

Evaluation

See Program Requirements for the Subspecialties of Diagnostic Radiology for evaluation requirements.

6 PROGRAM REQUIREMENTS FOR RESIDENCY EDUCATION IN MUSCULOSKELETAL RADIOLOGY

In addition to complying with the Program Requirements for Residency Education in the Subspecialties of Diagnostic Radiology, programs must comply with the following requirements, which in some cases may exceed the common requirements.

Scope and Duration of Training

DEFINITION AND SCOPE OF THE SUBSPECIALTY

The musculoskeletal radiology training program constitutes a closely supervised experience in the application and interpretation of all imaging examinations and procedures as they relate to the analysis of disorders of the musculoskeletal system, including bones, joints, and soft tissues. The imaging methods and procedures include, but are not necessarily limited to, routine radiography, computed tomography, ultrasonography, radionuclide scintigraphy, magnetic resonance, arthrography, and image-guided percutaneous biopsy techniques. The objective of training in musculoskeletal radiology is to provide an organized, comprehensive, supervised, and progressively responsible full-time educational experience in the selection,

interpretation, and performance of these examinations and procedures. A further objective is to provide the resident an opportunity to develop skills necessary for clinical and/or basic research in the subspecialty of musculoskeletal radiology.

DURATION OF TRAINING

The program shall offer 1 year of graduate medical education in musculoskeletal radiology. Completion of an ACGME-accredited program in diagnostic radiology or its equivalent must precede the period of training in musculoskeletal radiology.

Faculty Qualifications and Responsibilities

The program director must be certified in diagnostic radiology or radiology by the American Board of Radiology or possess equivalent qualifications.

In addition to the program director, the program must include at least one person experienced in musculoskeletal radiology who has a substantial commitment to the training program. If necessary, other radiologists with expertise in certain imaging methods or procedures may function at least as part-

Source: ACGME, February 1996; effective, February 1996. *Graduate Medical Education Directory, 2001–2002.* American Medical Association.

time members of the training program. To ensure adequate supervision of the residents, there must be at least one full-time faculty person available for each two residents in the program.

Facilities and Resources
SPACE AND EQUIPMENT

Modern facilities and equipment and adequate space must be available to ensure an adequate educational experience for the resident. Access to routine radiographic, computed tomographic, scintigraphic, magnetic resonance, and ultrasound equipment must be provided. Adequate space for film display, film interpretation, and consultation with referring physicians must be available, and adequate office space, office supplies, and secretarial help for the conduct of research projects should be provided for musculoskeletal radiology faculty and residents. Assistance with literature searches, editing, statistical tabulation, and photography should be provided.

LIBRARY

The training program must provide ancillary teaching resources including access to a medical library with a sufficient number of textbooks and journals related to musculoskeletal diseases and electronic literature search capabilities. A musculoskeletal radiology/pathology teaching file must be developed and available for use by the residents. The American College of Radiology teaching file will only partially meet this requirement.

Educational Program
CLINICAL COMPONENTS

Residents in musculoskeletal radiology must be provided access to a variety of patients encompassing the entire range of disorders of the musculoskeletal system, including articular, degenerative, metabolic, hematopoietic, infectious, traumatic, vascular, congenital, and neoplastic diseases. The imaging methods and procedures available for training should include routine radiography, computed tomography, ultrasonography, radionuclide scintigraphy, magnetic resonance, arthrography, and image-guided percutaneous biopsy techniques.

The program curriculum must provide clinical experience and didactic sessions encompassing the entire spectrum of musculoskeletal diseases. This must include both the axial and the appendicular skeletons of both adult and pediatric patients. The resident must interpret, under appropriate supervision, diagnostic examinations that include routine radiography, computed tomography, and magnetic resonance. Furthermore, the resident must perform and interpret arthrograms. The program must provide experience with image-guided percutaneous biopsy procedures and exposure to ultrasonography, bone densitometry, and radionuclide scintigraphy as they relate to diseases of the musculoskeletal system. A log must be kept by each resident documenting the types of arthrographic and biopsy procedures that she or he performs. With regard to invasive procedures, residents are to be given graduated responsibility as competence increases; such responsibility should include preprocedural and postprocedural patient care. Emphasis is placed on close coordination and cooperation with referring physicians, including orthopedic surgeons, rheumatologists, and emergency department specialists, and on establishment of proper imaging protocols to ensure that excessive or inappropriate examinations are not ordered and performed. Access to both inpatients and outpatients is required.

DIDACTIC COMPONENTS

There must be didactic conferences and teaching sessions that provide coverage of musculoskeletal concepts related to anatomy, physiology, pathology, orthopedic surgery, and rheumatology. Attendance at and participation in department conferences such as daily film interpretation sessions are required. Regularly scheduled interdepartmental conferences in, for example, orthopedic surgery, neurosurgery, and other appropriate surgical specialties (as well as pathology, rheumatology, and oncology) are also necessary components of the program. In addition, the training experience should include radiology-oriented conferences with medical students and graduate medical staff. The resident also should be encouraged to attend at least one national meeting or postgraduate course dealing with musculoskeletal radiology during his or her fellowship year.

Although the precise responsibility of the resident will vary from one clinical conference to another, opportunities must exist for active participation in the formulation of a diagnosis and/or the generation of an imaging protocol; such participation is to be used as a means by which the program director and other faculty members judge the resident's progress.

RESIDENT PARTICIPATION IN RESEARCH

The training period in musculoskeletal radiology should provide sufficient research opportunities for the resident. He or she should be able to participate in the design, performance, and interpretation of research studies and have the opportunity to develop competence in critical assessment of investigative techniques. Completion of at least one clinical or basic research investigation during the period of training is encouraged. Laboratory facilities to support research projects should be available in the institution.

INTERCHANGE WITH RESIDENTS IN OTHER SPECIALTIES

The presence of accredited training programs in orthopedic surgery and rheumatology is highly desirable.

Shared experiences with residents in orthopedic surgery, rheumatology, pathology, and other appropriate specialties, including surgical subspecialties, are strongly encouraged. When appropriate, supervision and teaching by faculty expert in these additional disciplines should be available.

Evaluation

See Program Requirements for Residency Education in the Subspecialties of Diagnostic Radiology for details concerning evaluation requirements.

7 PROGRAM REQUIREMENTS FOR RESIDENCY EDUCATION IN NEURORADIOLOGY

In addition to complying with the Program Requirements for Residency Education in the Subspecialties of Diagnostic Radiology, programs must comply with the following requirements, which may in some cases exceed the common requirements.

Scope and Duration of Training

DEFINITION AND SCOPE OF THE SUBSPECIALTY

The body of knowledge and practice of neuroradiology comprises both imaging and interventional procedures related to the brain, spine and spinal cord, head, neck, and organs of special sense in adults and children. Special training and skills are required to enable the neuroradiologist to function as an expert diagnostic and therapeutic consultant and practitioner. The objective of training in this subspecialty of radiology is to provide residents with an organized, comprehensive, and highly supervised full-time educational experience in the selection, interpretation, and performance of these examinations and procedures and to provide them with opportunities and skills for research in the field of neuroradiology.

DURATION OF TRAINING

The program shall offer 1 year of graduate medical education in neuroradiology. This year of training must follow successful completion of an ACGME-accredited program in diagnostic radiology or its equivalent.

Faculty Qualifications and Responsibilities

The program director shall have had appropriate postresidency experience in neuroradiology, preferably fellowship training.

At a minimum, the neuroradiology faculty must include, in addition to the program director, one or more neuroradiologists whose total time commitment to neuroradiology is at least one half-time equivalent and who are able to devote adequate time to the program. Their expertise may be limited to a segment of neuroradiology or a related discipline, e.g., interventional neuroradiology, pediatric neuroradiology, or head and neck radiology. The faculty must provide didactic teaching and supervision of the residents' performance and interpretations of neuroradiologic procedures. The minimum number of residents need not be greater than one, but two residents are desirable. To ensure adequate supervision and evaluation of a resident's academic progress, the faculty/resident ratio should not be less than one full-time faculty person for every two residents.

Facilities and Resources

SPACE AND EQUIPMENT

The following equipment, which should be "state of the art," should be available: magnetic resonance imaging, computed tomography, film-screen and digital subtraction angiography (DSA), a radiographic-fluoroscopic room(s) with tilt table suitable for performing myelography, and conventional radiographic and tomographic equipment. The examination rooms should be equipped for monitoring so that examinations may be performed in high-risk patients. Adjacent to or within examination rooms there should be facilities for storing the catheters, gowns, embolic materials, contrast material, and other supplies needed for the conduct of neuroradiologic procedures. A room should be available near the angiographic room for sterilization and preparation of catheters, instrument trays, and other reusable supplies. There must be adequate space within the department to house these facilities.

Adequate areas for film display, interpretation of films, and consultation with clinicians must be available. There must be adequate office space and support space for neuroradiology faculty/staff and residents.

The program should provide office space, office supplies, and secretarial help for the conduct of research projects. Assistance with literature searches, editing, statistical tabulation, and photography should be provided.

LABORATORY

The institution should provide laboratory facilities to support research projects. It is highly desirable to have an animal facility with radiographic-fluoroscopic equipment, particularly that which might be used for invasive diagnostic and therapeutic neuroradiologic procedures.

LIBRARY

There should be ready access to a library of general medical texts and periodicals. In particular, there should be periodicals and texts in the fields of neuroradiology, diagnostic radiology, head and neck radiology, neurology, neurosurgery, neuroanatomy, and orthopedic surgery. It is desirable that computerized literature search facilities also be available.

Educational Program

CURRICULUM

The program must offer the opportunity for residents to perform, consult, conduct, and interpret (under close supervision), invasive as well as noninvasive procedures in neuroradiology. The procedures shall include cerebral angiography, myelography, computed tomography, magnetic resonance imaging, ultrasound of the central nervous system and vessels, and plain film radiography related to the brain, head, neck, and spine. It is also desirable that there be exposure to positron emission tomography (PET) and magnetic resonance spectroscopy. With

Source: ACGME, February 1990; effective, July 1995. *Graduate Medical Education Directory, 2001–2002*, American Medical Association.

regard to invasive procedures, residents must be given graduated responsibility in the performance of the procedures as competence increases. Responsibility for these procedures should include preprocedural and postprocedural patient care.

CLINICAL COMPONENTS

Clinical and educational experience in the basic clinical neurosciences, e.g., neurosurgery, neurology, neuropathology, neuro-otolaryngology, and neuro-ophthalmology, and in the basic radiologic sciences, e.g., radiation and magnetic resonance physics, radiation biology, and the pharmacology of radiographic contrast materials, must be provided. It is expected that there will be strong clinical services in neurologic surgery and neurology in the institution sponsoring the neuroradiology program. Most the time in the program should be spent in clinical training in neuroradiology.

The program in neuroradiology must provide a sufficient volume and variety of patients with neurologic, neurosurgical, neuro-ophthalmologic, neuro-otorhinolaryngologic, spinal, and other pertinent disorders so that residents gain adequate experience in the full gamut of neuroradiologic examinations, procedures, and interpretations. The program must provide an adequate volume and variety of invasive procedures (e.g., neuroangiography, myelography, DSA, and therapeutic embolization) and noninvasive neuroradiologic examinations (e.g., computed tomography, magnetic resonance, and plain film studies). The program director should require residents to maintain documentation of the invasive cases in which they have been the performing radiologist and should review the logs with them at least once in the course of the training year. Clinical experience may be supplemented by training through affiliations with other institutions.

DIDACTIC COMPONENTS

There shall be intradepartmental conferences as well as conferences with related clinical departments in which residents and residents participate on a regular basis. These should include one or more weekly departmental conferences in neuroradiology, as well as institutional conferences in clinical neu-

rosciences that are held at least monthly. Residents should be encouraged to attend and participate in local extramural conferences and should attend at least one national meeting or postgraduate course in neuroradiology while in training.

Residents should be encouraged to present the radiologic aspects of cases that are discussed in clinical conferences related to the allied disciplines, such as neurosurgery and the neurologic sciences. They should also prepare clinically or pathologically proven cases for inclusion in the teaching file.

There should be daily "film reading" conferences that should require residents to reach their own diagnostic conclusions, which should then be reviewed and criticized by faculty/staff. These conferences need not be limited to clinically current cases, but may be based on cases that are already within the teaching file. Diagnostic reports generated by residents should be closely reviewed for content, level of confidence, grammar, and style.

RESIDENT PARTICIPATION IN RESEARCH

Residents should be encouraged to undertake investigative study of either a clinical or basic science nature. At least one project of such merit that it could be submitted for publication should be encouraged.

INTERCHANGE WITH RESIDENTS IN OTHER SPECIALTIES AND STUDENTS

Residents should be encouraged to participate in the research projects of residents and staff persons in other specialties. They should attend clinical conferences in other specialties and serve as consultants to these conferences. It is desirable that they participate in the clinical teaching of medical students and also in the preclinical curriculum in subjects such as anatomy and physiology.

Evaluation

See Program Requirements for Residency Education in the Subspecialties of Diagnostic Radiology for details concerning evaluation requirements.

8 PROGRAM REQUIREMENTS FOR RESIDENCY EDUCATION IN NUCLEAR RADIOLOGY

In addition to complying with the Program Requirements for Residency Education in the Subspecialties of Diagnostic Radiology, programs must comply with the following requirements, which may in some cases exceed the common requirements.

Scope and Duration of Training

DEFINITION AND SCOPE OF THE SPECIALTY

Nuclear radiology is defined as a clinical subspecialty of radiology involving imaging by external detection of radionuclides and/or biodistribution by external detection of radionuclides in the body for diagnosis of disease. Residency training programs in nuclear radiology must provide advanced training in the medical uses of radionuclides for in vivo imaging.

A training program in nuclear radiology will be accredited only in those institutions that have an accredited training program in diagnostic radiology.

A program in nuclear radiology will be reviewed and accredited in conjunction with the review and accreditation of the residency program in diagnostic radiology.

DURATION OF TRAINING

The program shall offer 1 year of graduate medical education in nuclear radiology. The year of training must follow successful completion of an ACGME-accredited residency program in diagnostic radiology or its equivalent.

Institutional Organization

Those aspects of institutional support that pertain to residencies in diagnostic radiology shall also apply to programs in nuclear radiology, e.g., administrative support, facilities, and clinical resources.

Faculty Qualifications and Responsibilities

The program director is responsible for the instructional program and for supervision of residents. The program director shall be certified by the American Board of Radiology with Special Competence in Nuclear Radiology or by the American Board of Nuclear Medicine or possess suitable equivalent qualifications. It is desirable that faculty members be certified in boards appropriate to those areas in which they are assigned to instruct and supervise residents. They must contribute sufficient time to the program to provide adequate instruction and supervision.

A faculty (nuclear medicine physician)/resident ratio of 1:2 should adequately provide for teaching and supervisory responsibilities.

Facilities and Resources

State-of-the-art nuclear imaging equipment should be available for instructional purposes.

Educational Program

The educational program must provide for well-balanced and progressive resident participation through examination of a diverse patient population, with continuous teaching and an active research effort in nuclear radiology.

CLINICAL COMPONENT

1. The training program shall include graduated study, experience, and responsibility in all facets of nuclear radiologic diagnosis, medical nuclear and diagnostic radiologic physics, radiobiology, health physics and protection, nuclear medical instrumentation, radiopharmaceutical chemistry and instrumentation, clinical applications of nuclear radiology, and pathology.
2. The program must provide adequate opportunity for a resident to participate in and personally perform a broad range of nuclear radiologic procedures.

DIDACTIC COMPONENTS

1. Formal instruction in diagnostic radiologic and medical nuclear physics, radiobiology, and radiopharmaceutical chemistry is required.
2. Appropriate emphasis must be placed on the educational value of teaching rounds and conferences. In addition, there should be frequent interdepartmental teaching conferences.

RESEARCH

The program should provide an environment in which a resident is encouraged to engage in investigative work with appropriate faculty supervision. Documentation of this environment should be made in the application and indicated by papers published by residents and/or clinical faculty.

TEACHING FILE

A teaching file of images referable to all aspects of nuclear radiology must be available for use by residents. This file should be indexed, coded, and currently maintained.

Evaluation

See Program Requirements for Residency Education in the Subspecialties of Diagnostic Radiology for details concerning evaluation requirements.

Source: ACGME, September 1996; effective, July 1997. *Graduate Medical Education Directory, 2001–2002*, American Medical Association.

9 PROGRAM REQUIREMENTS FOR RESIDENCY EDUCATION IN PEDIATRIC RADIOLOGY

In addition to complying with the Program Requirements for Residency Education in the Subspecialties of Diagnostic Radiology, programs must comply with the following requirements, which may in some cases exceed the common requirements.

Scope and Duration of Training

DEFINITION AND SCOPE OF THE SPECIALTY

The training program in the subspecialty of pediatric radiology constitutes a supervised experience in the pediatric applications and interpretation of radiography, computed tomography, ultrasonography, angiography, interventional techniques, nuclear radiology, magnetic resonance, and any other imaging modality customarily included within the specialty of diagnostic radiology.

The program should be structured to enhance substantially the resident's knowledge of the applications of all forms of diagnostic imaging to the unique clinical/pathophysiologic problems of the newborn, infant, child, and adolescent. The fundamentals of radiobiology, radiologic physics, and radiation protection as they relate to the infant, child, and adolescent should be reviewed during the pediatric radiology training experience. The program must provide residents direct and progressively responsible experience in pediatric imaging as they advance through training. This training must culminate in sufficiently independent responsibility for clinical decision making such that the program ensures that the graduating resident has achieved the ability to execute sound clinical judgment.

DURATION OF TRAINING

The program shall offer 1 year of graduate medical education in pediatric radiology. Completion of an ACGME-accredited program in diagnostic radiology or its equivalent must precede advanced training in pediatric radiology.

OBJECTIVES AND GOALS

The educational program in pediatric radiology shall meet training objectives so that on completion of the program the resident is able to:

1. Understand the developmental and acquired disease processes of the newborn, infant, child, and adolescent, which are basic to the practice of pediatric and adolescent medicine.
2. Perform and interpret radiologic and imaging studies of the pediatric patient.
3. Supervise and teach the elements of radiography and radiology as they pertain to infants and children
4. Understand how to design and perform research (clinical, biomedical, educational, health services).

Institutional Organization

A program of pediatric radiology training should function whenever feasible in direct association and/or affiliation with an ACGME-accredited program in diagnostic radiology. Pediatric radiology programs may be conducted in either a children's hospital or a general hospital.

Faculty Qualifications and Responsibilities

PROGRAM DIRECTOR

The program director must have sufficient academic and administrative experience to ensure effective implementation of these program requirements and should have had at least 5 years of participation as an active faculty member in an accredited pediatric radiology program. The program director must be certified by the American Board of Radiology in radiology or diagnostic radiology or possess equivalent qualifications. The program director must have received the Certificate of Added Qualifications in Pediatric Radiology granted by the American Board of Radiology or possess equivalent qualifications. The director must devote sufficient time to the program to fulfill all the responsibilities inherent in meeting the educational goals of the program. The program director is responsible for establishing the curriculum as well as procedures for evaluation of the resident's competency. Periodic evaluation of the resident with feedback is required. The program director shall select and supervise the trainees and shall select pediatric radiology program faculty members.

FACULTY

There should be sufficient qualified professional personnel to constitute a teaching faculty. The faculty should comprise no fewer than three experienced radiologists, including the program director, who work full-time in pediatric radiology and its related subspecialty areas and are able to devote adequate time to the program. The minimum faculty requirement may be met by the program director and two other full-time equivalent (i.e., a total of three or more individuals) faculty members. Although it is desirable that pediatric radiologists supervise special imaging (i.e., angiography, interventional radiology, nuclear radiology, computed tomography, magnetic resonance), when they are not expert in an imaging technique, other radiologists who are specialists in that imaging method should be part-time members of the pediatric radiology faculty. Because such radiologists are usually not broadly experienced in the discipline and practice of pediatric radiology, pediatric radiologists should participate in the interpretation and correlation of the findings of these special imaging examinations.

Source: ACGME, September 1997; effective, July 1998. Graduate Medical Education Directory, 2001–2002. American Medical Association.

A ratio of at least two pediatric radiologists for every resident is essential to provide adequate opportunity for teaching and supervision.

Facilities and Resources
SPACE AND EQUIPMENT
Modern facilities and equipment in adequate space must be available and functioning to accomplish the overall educational program in pediatric radiology. Diagnostic imaging modalities shall include radiography, computed tomography, ultrasonography, radionuclide scintigraphy, angiography, and magnetic resonance imaging. The department must have a minimum of one radiographic/fluoroscopic room, one ultrasound unit, one angiographic room, one computed tomography scanner, one magnetic resonance imaging unit, and one nuclear radiology gamma camera. All equipment must be up to date. There must be justification for continued use of any equipment that is more than 10 years of age.

In general hospitals that treat patients of all ages, pediatric radiology is often a section of the radiology department; similarly, special imaging services of such departments are separate sections. In such cases, there should be recognition within the special imaging sections of the particular needs of the pediatric radiology program. There should be low-dose roentgenographic/fluoroscopic facilities specifically for children. The availability of all special imaging services for pediatric radiology residents is essential.

Laboratory and pathology services must be adequate to permit residents to enhance their educational experience during the diagnostic imaging and care of patients and to obtain timely correlation with diagnostic imaging studies.

INPATIENT AND OUTPATIENT SERVICES
The hospital must have sufficient inpatient and outpatient services in general and subspecialty pediatrics to ensure a broad, in-depth exposure to pediatrics. The pediatric clinical services must be part of the teaching program and should require diagnostic imaging input for many of their patients.

LIBRARY
Learning resources should include access to an institutional and/or departmental library with current journals and textbooks sufficient to cover the specialty of pediatrics and pediatric subspecialties, radiology, and related fields. The library must contain journals and current textbooks on all aspects of pediatric radiology. The institutional library must have a librarian and facilities for electronic database searches. Moreover, the methods of performing such electronic database searches must be taught to residents. A pediatric radiology teaching file must be available for use by pediatric radiology residents. This teaching file should contain a minimum of 500 cases that are indexed, coded, actively maintained, and continually enhanced with new cases. Availability of the American College of Radiology pediatric learning file or its equivalent is desirable; this only partially meets the teaching file requirements.

PATIENT POPULATION
There should be an ACGME-accredited residency in pediatrics, as well as pediatric medical and surgical subspecialty programs, to provide an appropriate patient population and educational resources in the institution. In addition to full-time pediatricians, there should be one or more pediatric surgeons, one or more pediatric pathologists, and a broad range of pediatric medical and surgical subspecialists.

The institution's pediatric population must include patients with a diversity of pediatric illnesses from which broad experience can be gained. The number of pediatric radiology residents in a program at any given time should reflect the patient census to ensure each trainee of an adequate experience. The program must have sufficient volume and variety of patients to ensure that residents gain experience in the full range of pediatric radiologic examinations, procedures, and interpretations. A reasonable experience is no less than 15,000 pediatric radiologic examinations per year per resident.

Educational Program
CURRICULUM
The training should consist of didactic and clinical experiences that encompass the scope of pediatric radiology from the neonate to the adolescent. Every organ system should be studied in the contexts of growth and development, congenital malformations, diseases peculiar to infants and children, and diseases beginning in childhood but causing substantial residual impairment in adulthood. The didactic component should promote scholarship, self-instruction, self-evaluation, teaching, and research activity. It should foster the development of analytic skills and judgment. The clinical component should facilitate skillful technical performance of low radiation dose procedures on all organ systems that are examined in the practice of pediatric radiology. The pediatric imaging experience should include both inpatient and outpatient studies.

Residents must have graded responsibility and supervision in the performance of procedures and the perfection of technical and interpretive skills. It is essential that the pediatric radiology trainee be instructed in common pediatric imaging technical procedures and their indications, limitations, judicious utilization, and risks, including radiation dose considerations. The pediatric radiology resident must also be instructed in the risks and benefits of pediatric sedation; this includes an understanding of the physician's role in the monitoring and management of pediatric patients during and after sedation for diagnostic and therapeutic procedures. When the program is conducted in a general hospital, the pediatric radiology trainee must have training in imaging examinations of pediatric patients.

The scope of a 1-year training program in pediatric radiology shall include all diagnostic imaging applicable to the pediatric patient. The 1-year training program should include no more than 4 weeks of vacation. The curriculum must include the central nervous, musculoskeletal, cardiopulmonary, gastrointestinal, and genitourinary systems. In each organ system, the effective and appropriate use of imaging modalities, including ultrasound, computed tomography, magnetic resonance, nuclear radiology, and vascular/interventional radiology, should be taught. The resident is responsible for following the imaging workup of the patient and must be substantially involved in the performance and interpretation of examinations that utilize various modalities. Correlation of radiologic findings with the clinical management and outcome of the pediatric patient is essential.

CLINICAL COMPONENT

The pediatric radiology training program should provide a minimum number of procedures available per year per resident as follows:

300 fluoroscopic procedures

300 ultrasound examinations

200 body imaging (computed tomography/magnetic resonance) examinations

The number of these procedures available for the pediatric radiology resident should not have an adverse impact on the education of the diagnostic radiology residents in the same institution.

The pediatric radiology resident must have at least 3 weeks of experience in each of the following specialized areas: pediatric neuroradiology, vascular/interventional radiology, and nuclear radiology. This experience may be obtained through a combination of lectures, conferences, seminars, and involvement as the primary or secondary operator and by observing procedures. Supervised instruction should be provided by physicians with special expertise in those disciplines. It is acceptable to supplement the pediatric experience with adult patients in some specialties, such as vascular and interventional radiology, to enhance teaching. The program must require that residents maintain a logbook and document their training in nuclear radiology, neuroradiology, and vascular/interventional radiology. The logbook should include the patient name, medical record number, and procedure(s) performed. The minimum numbers of procedures per resident performed in these specialized areas of pediatric radiology are as follows:

50 pediatric nuclear radiology studies

200 neuroimaging studies

25 vascular/interventional studies

Residents in pediatric radiology should serve as pediatric radiologic consultants with the supervision and mentoring of faculty pediatric radiologists. The teaching experience should include conferences oriented toward pediatrics and radiology with medical students, residents, medical staff, and health care professionals.

DIDACTIC COMPONENT

Study of clinical and basic sciences as they relate to radiology and pediatrics shall be a part of the didactic program. Subspecialty conferences, seminars, and academic review activities

in pediatric radiology must be regularly scheduled. It is essential that the resident participate in the planning and presenting of conferences. In addition to conferences, study is integrated with the performance and interpretation of roentgenographic and other imaging examinations.

Residents must attend a minimum of three departmental conferences per week dedicated to pediatric radiology and participate in three or more interdepartmental conferences or rounds per week. When attending the conferences of other specialties (for example, tumor board, morbidity and mortality, and surgery conferences), the pediatric residents should present the radiographic portions of the conferences. The resident must be involved in daily radiology working conferences (daily conferences reviewing radiographs of intensive care units, other inpatient teams, and so forth). In the course of the 12-month program, residents should attend and participate in at least 20 teaching conferences, such as grand rounds, sponsored by pediatric subspecialty departments. A journal club or research club must meet monthly.

RESIDENT POLICIES

Supervision

The responsibility or independence given to residents should depend on their knowledge, skills, and experience. Additional personnel must be available within an appropriate time interval to perform or to supervise procedures.

Duty Hours and Conditions of Work

Duty hours and night and weekend call for trainees must reflect responsibility for patients and provide for adequate patient care. Residents must not be required regularly to perform excessively difficult or prolonged duties. It is the responsibility of the program director to ensure assignment of reasonable in-hospital duty hours. Residents who are taking night or weekend call must always have assigned faculty who are available for on-call coverage.

OTHER REQUIRED COMPONENTS

Resident Participation in Research

The training program in pediatric radiology should have a research component that will offer the resident an opportunity to learn the fundamentals of design, performance, interpretation of research studies, and evaluation of investigative methods. Trainees should develop competence in critical assessment of imaging research, patient outcome data, and the scientific literature.

The resident should participate in clinical, basic biomedical, or health services research projects and submit at least one scientific paper or exhibit to a regional or national meeting. The resident should participate in the quality improvement program of the department.

Appointment of Other Residents

The training program should have close interaction with a diagnostic radiology residency. Shared experience with residents in general pediatrics and in the pediatric-related subspecialties, i.e., surgery, pathology, and cardiology, is strongly encouraged;

when appropriate, supervision and teaching by expert faculty in these disciplines should occur. The resident must also be involved in teaching conferences for medical students, radiology residents, other residents rotating on the pediatric radiology service, and other health professional training programs.

The subspecialty program in pediatric radiology must not have an adverse impact, such as by dilution of the available clinical material, on the education of the diagnostic radiology residents in the same institution.

Evaluation

The RRC will consider as one measure of a program's quality the performance of its graduates on the examination of the American Board of Radiology for the Certificate of Added Qualifications in Pediatric Radiology. All program graduates should take the examination (*see* Program Requirements for Residency Education in the Subspecialties of Diagnostic Radiology for additional evaluation requirements).

10 PROGRAM REQUIREMENTS FOR RESIDENCY EDUCATION IN VASCULAR AND INTERVENTIONAL RADIOLOGY

In addition to complying with the Program Requirements for Residency Education in the Subspecialties of Diagnostic Radiology, programs must comply with the following requirements, which in some cases exceed the common requirements.

Scope and Duration of Training
DEFINITION AND SCOPE OF THE SPECIALTY

The unique clinical and invasive nature of practice in vascular and interventional radiology requires special training and skills. The educational program in the subspecialty of vascular and interventional radiology must be organized to provide comprehensive, full-time training and experience in the evaluation and management of patients requiring imaging guided diagnostic vascular and interventional procedures and a supervised experience in the performance of image-guided diagnostic methods of treating disease. Vascular and interventional procedures are guided by a number of imaging modalities, including fluoroscopy, angiography, computed tomography, ultrasonography, magnetic resonance imaging, radionuclide scintigraphy, and other modalities included within the specialty of radiology. The training program must be structured to enhance substantially the resident's knowledge of the application of all forms of imaging to the performance and interpretation of vascular and interventional procedures.

The program in vascular and interventional radiology must be structured to enhance the resident's knowledge of the signs and symptoms of disorders amenable to diagnosis and/or treatment by percutaneous techniques. The significance of the symptoms must be understood, as well as the pathophysiology and natural history of the disorders. Residents must know the indications for and contraindications to vascular and interventional procedures and understand the medical and surgical alternatives to those procedures. The vascular and interventional radiologist must have a complete understanding of imaging methods used to guide percutaneous procedures. The resident must become skilled in the technical aspects of percutaneous proce-

dures. The fundamentals of radiation physics, radiation biology, and radiation protection should all be reviewed during the vascular and interventional training experience. In addition, training should provide opportunities for research into new technologies and evaluation of the clinical outcomes of interventional radiology.

DURATION OF TRAINING

The program shall offer 1 year of graduate medical education in vascular and interventional radiology. This year of training must follow successful completion of an ACGME-accredited program in diagnostic radiology or its equivalent.

FACULTY/RESIDENT NUMBERS

The minimum number of residents is one. To ensure an adequate educational experience as well as adequate supervision and evaluation of a resident's academic progress, the faculty/resident ratio must not be less than one full-time faculty person for every resident.

Program Director/Faculty
PROGRAM DIRECTOR

The program director must be certified by the American Board of Radiology in diagnostic radiology or radiology and have a Certificate of Added Qualifications in Vascular and Interventional Radiology from the American Board of Radiology or possess equivalent qualifications.

FACULTY

There should be sufficient qualified professional personnel to constitute a teaching faculty. The faculty should comprise at least two full-time vascular and interventional radiologists, including the program director. Although the expertise of any one faculty member may be limited to a particular aspect of vascular and interventional radiology, the training program must

Source: ACGME, June 22, 1998; effective, July 1, 1999. *Graduates Medical Education Directory, 2001–2002*, American Medical Association

provide experience that includes all aspects of vascular and nonvascular interventional radiology. The faculty must provide didactic teaching and direct supervision of residents' performance in the clinical patient management, procedural, interpretative, and consultative aspects of vascular and interventional radiology. The faculty must demonstrate a commitment to the subspecialty of vascular interventional radiology. Such commitment includes membership in professional societies, publications in the field, and/or a minimum of 30 hours of CME Category I credit per year (*see* Program Requirements for the Subspecialties of Diagnostic Radiology for additional program director and faculty requirements).

Facilities and Resources

SPACE AND EQUIPMENT

Modern imaging/procedure rooms and equipment in adequate space must be available to permit the performance of all vascular and interventional radiologic procedures. Imaging modalities in the department should include fluoroscopy, angiography, computed tomography, ultrasonography, magnetic resonance imaging, and radionuclide scintigraphy. Fluoroscopic equipment should be high resolution and have digital display with postprocedure image processing capability. Rooms in which vascular and interventional procedures are performed must be equipped with physiologic monitoring and resuscitative equipment. Suitable recovery and patient holding areas should be available. Adjacent to or within procedure rooms, there should be facilities for storing catheters, guidewires, contrast materials, embolic agents, and other supplies. There must be adequate space and facilities for image display, image interpretation, and consultation with other clinicians. There must be adequate office space and support space for vascular and interventional radiology faculty or staff and residents.

PATIENT POPULATION

The institution's patient population must have a diversity of illnesses from which a broad experience in vascular and interventional radiology can be obtained. There must also be an adequate variety and number of interventional procedures for each resident. Each resident must document his or her direct participation in a minimum of 500 vascular and interventional procedures that cover the entire range of the specialty. The procedures should be recorded in a personal case log that should be reviewed periodically with the program director. Clinical experience may be supplemented by training affiliations to other institutions.

LIBRARY

Teaching resources must include a medical library with access to a variety of textbooks and journals in radiology, vascular and interventional radiology, and related fields. A coded vascular and interventional radiology teaching film file is desirable. The resident should have access to computerized literature search facilities.

SUPPORT SERVICES

Pathology and medical laboratory services and consultation must be regularly and conveniently available to meet the needs of patients, as determined by the medical staff. Services should be available each day throughout the entire 24 hours. At least one qualified medical technologist must be on duty or available at all times. Diagnostic laboratories for the noninvasive assessment of peripheral vascular disease also must be available. Nursing support should be readily available, particularly if conscious sedation might be administered.

RESEARCH FACILITIES

The institution should provide laboratory and ancillary facilities to support research projects. These laboratory facilities and research opportunities may be made available to vascular and interventional radiology residents through cooperative arrangements with other departments or institutions.

The Educational Program

CLINICAL COMPONENTS

The training program curriculum must include didactic and clinical experiences that encompass the full clinical spectrum of vascular and interventional radiology. Residents must have the opportunity to carry out all of the following under close, graded responsibility and supervision: clinical preprocedure evaluation of patients, interpretation of preliminary diagnostic studies, consultation with clinicians on other services, performance of vascular and interventional procedures, generation of procedural reports, and delivery of both short- and long-term follow-up care. The continuity of care must be of sufficient duration to enable the resident to obtain appropriate feedback regarding the management of patients under his or her care.

Both vascular and nonvascular interventional procedures, excluding the intracerebral vascular system, must be included in the training program. Examples of vascular procedures include but are not limited to arteriography, venography, lymphography, angioplasty and related percutaneous revascularization procedures, embolotherapy, transcatheter infusion therapy, intravascular foreign body removal, and percutaneous placement of endovascular prostheses such as stent grafts and inferior vena cava filters and insertion of vascular access devices and catheters. Examples of nonvascular procedures include, but are not limited to, percutaneous imaging-guided biopsy; percutaneous gastrostomy; percutaneous nephrostomy; ureteral stenting and other transcatheter genitourinary procedures for diagnosis and for treatment of lithiasis, obstruction, and fistula; percutaneous transhepatic and transcholecystic biliary procedures; percutaneous drainage for diagnosis and treatment of infections and other fluid collections; and miscellaneous percutaneous imaging-guided procedures such as ablation of neoplasms and cysts. Residents must have specific clinical time dedicated to the performance and interpretation of vascular ultrasound studies, magnetic resonance angiograms, and computed tomography angiograms.

The responsibility or independence given to residents must depend on an assessment of their knowledge, manual skill, and experience. In supervising residents during vascular and interventional procedures, faculty members should reinforce the understanding gained during residency training of X-ray generators, image intensifiers, film, screen-film combinations, film changers, film processing, ultrasonography, computed tomography, and other imaging modalities. Residents must be provided with instruction in the use of needles, catheters, and guidewires and must be directly supervised and given graduated responsibility in the performance of procedures as competence increases. A thorough understanding of the clinical indications, risks, interpretation, and limitations of vascular and interventional procedures is essential to the practice of vascular and interventional radiology. Residents must be instructed in these areas.

Residents should also be instructed in proper use and interpretation of laboratory tests and in methods that are adjunctive to vascular and interventional procedures, such as use of physiologic monitoring devices, noninvasive vascular testing, and noninvasive vascular imaging. There should be specific instruction in the clinical aspects of patient assessment, patient treatment, planning, and patient management related to vascular and interventional radiology. There also should be instruction in the use of analgesics, antibiotics, and other drugs commonly employed in conjunction with these procedures. The residents must be thoroughly familiar with all aspects of administering and monitoring sedation of the conscious patient. They also must have advanced cardiac life support training.

Residents should serve as consultants under the supervision of staff vascular and interventional radiologists. Direct interactions of residents with patients must be closely observed to ensure that appropriate standards of care and concern for patient welfare are strictly maintained. Communication, consultation, and coordination of care with the referring clinical staff and clinical services must be maintained and documented with appropriate notes in the medical record. Reports for the medical record generated by residents should be closely reviewed by faculty for accuracy of content, grammar, style, and level of confidence. The vascular/interventional residents should also assist and train diagnostic radiology residents in the performance and interpretation of procedures.

DIDACTIC COMPONENTS

There shall be scheduled intradepartmental conferences as well as conferences with related clinical departments in which residents participate on a regular basis. These should include one or more specific weekly departmental conferences and at least one interdisciplinary conference per week at which attendance is required. In particular, interdepartmental conferences with the surgical specialties should be an important teaching component. The resident's teaching experience should include conferences with medical students, graduate medical staff, and allied health personnel. Scheduled presentations by the resident during these conferences should be encouraged.

Clinical and basic sciences as they relate to radiology and vascular and interventional radiology should be part of the didactic program. This should include but not be limited to the anatomy, physiology, and pathophysiology of the hematologic, circulatory, respiratory, gastrointestinal, genitourinary, and musculoskeletal systems. Relevant pharmacology, patient evaluation and management skills, and diagnostic techniques also should be addressed.

There must be documented regular review of all mortality and morbidity related to the performance of interventional procedures. Residents must participate actively in this review, which should be held not less than monthly. Residents should be encouraged to attend and participate in local extramural conferences and should attend at least one national meeting or postgraduate course in interventional radiology while in training. Participation in local or national vascular and interventional radiology societies should be encouraged. Residents should be encouraged to present the radiologic aspects of cases that are discussed in multidisciplinary conferences. They also should prepare clinically or pathologically proven cases for inclusion in the teaching file.

OTHER REQUIRED COMPONENTS
Resident Participation in Research

The residents should learn the fundamentals of experimental design, performance, and interpretation of results. They should participate in clinical, basic biomedical, or health services research projects and should be encouraged to undertake at least one project as principal investigator. They should submit at least one scientific paper or exhibit to a regional or national meeting. The opportunity also must be provided for residents to develop their competence in critical assessment of new imaging modalities and of new procedures in vascular and interventional radiology.

Scholarly Activity

See Program Requirements for Residency Education in the Subspecialties of Diagnostic Radiology for details concerning scholarly activity requirements.

Duty Hours and Conditions of Work

See Program Requirements for Residency Education in the Subspecialties of Diagnostic Radiology for details concerning duty hour requirements.

Evaluation

See Program Requirements for Residency Education in the Subspecialties of Diagnostic Radiology for details concerning evaluation requirements.

Board Certification

The Residency Review Committee will consider as one measure of a program's quality the performance of its graduates on the examination of the American Board of Radiology for the Certificate of Added Qualifications in Vascular Interventional Radiology. All program graduates should take the examination.